THE REBEL'S GUIDE TO RECOVERY

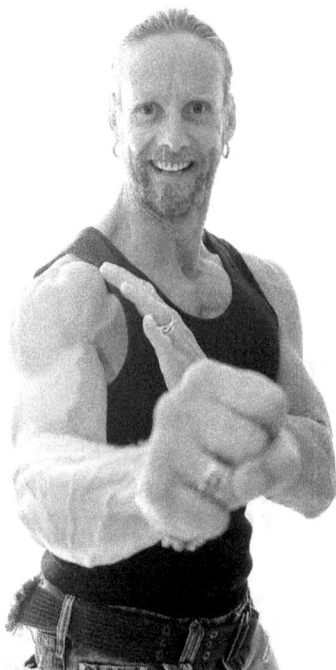

ABOUT THE AUTHOR

Born in Germany in 1958, and living in Australia since 1981, Jost is an ex speed-addict, dealer and deserter, turned drug and alcohol counselor who then became an acupuncturist. After lecturing in traditional Chinese medicine for a decade and running numerous health centres, he founded a holistic rehab based on his revolutionary recovery programs. Jost is also a media commentator, a columnist for health magazines and a speaker renowned for presenting his radical ideas about health in a highly entertaining manner.

www.jostsauer.com

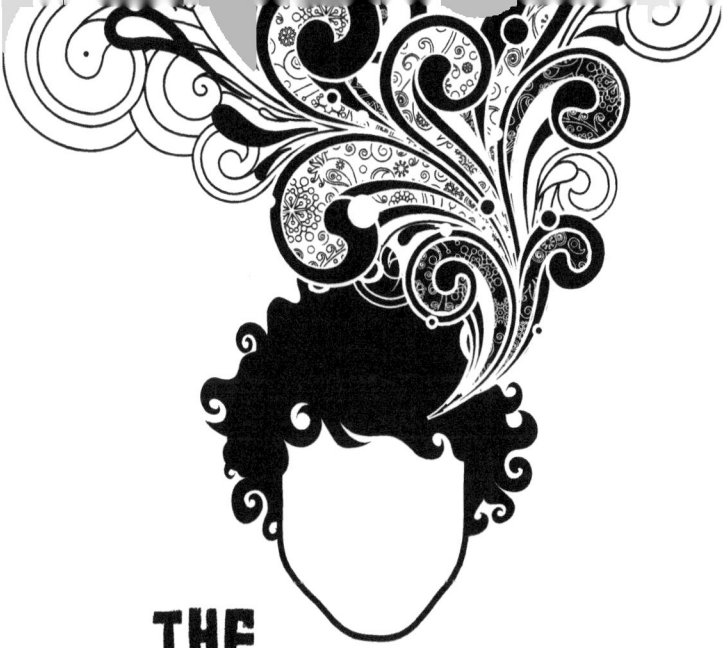

THE REBEL'S GUIDE TO RECOVERY

Jost Sauer

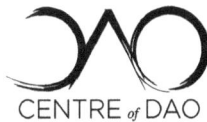

CENTRE *of* DAO

First published in 2014
Copyright © Jost Sauer 2014

Centre of Dao
21 Maple St
Maleny QLD 4552
Australia
info@centreofdao.com
+61 (0) 411 412 445

National Library of Australia Cataloguing-in-Publication entry

Creator: Sauer, Jost, author.

Title: The rebel's guide to recovery / Jost Sauer.

ISBN: 9780975725818 (paperback)

Subjects: Drug addiction--Treatment.
            Drug abuse--Treatment.
            Alcoholism--Treatment.
            Drug addicts--Rehabilitation.
            Alcoholics--Rehabilitation
            Medicine, Chinese.

Dewey Number: 616.8606

Design: Tony Giacca
Printed and bound in Australia by InHouse Print and Design
Published with the assistance of InHouse Publishing
www.inhousepublishing.com.au

for all the rebels

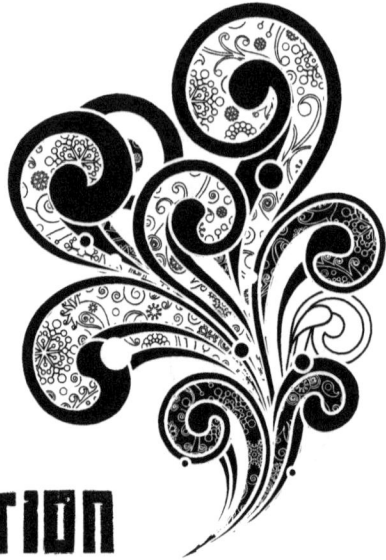

INTRODUCTION

In January 2011, I was speaking at an electronic music festival out in the country – as I often do – to one of the most laid-back audiences I've ever had. People were lying on the grass out the front of the marquee, listening while passing big joints around. Others lounged on the haystack seating, staring at the screen with glazed eyes or looking beatifically out-of-it. After the talk, the sound technician helped me pack up my equipment and carry it out the front of the tent. We stood for a moment looking over the festival site. It was late afternoon by then, the sky was a glowing sunset pink and the grass and trees looked intensely green. Music drifted on the air and groups of people in multicolored clothes were wandering through the tent village or dancing amongst the trees. The vibe was love and peace: 'Hobbiton on acid'.

I'd been talking about using past drug experiences as an evolutionary tool. The idea being that if millions of ex-drug users followed the path of self-realisation and sought to recapture altered states and consciousness expansion after drugs, the psychedelic revolution the hippies started would become psychedelic evolution, and there would no longer be a need for recreational drugs.

The sound tech said that he had really enjoyed my talk, then, looked out across the festival and asked, 'But how can I have all of this without drugs?' I chewed over his question as I walked back to my car. It was parked in a field full of shiny family cars; there was not a hippie vehicle in sight. The festival-goers were people who wanted to escape normal reality for a few days of substance-induced creativity, self-expression, music, bonding and bliss. But they would all be returning to 'reality' on Sunday night and then, more than likely, feeling a big come-down on Tuesday morning.

This is not how it's supposed to go. We are destined to live colorful, spontaneous and cosmically connected lives, and we are supposed to be expressive, eccentric, independent and uncaring of what the rest of society thinks of us, not just for three days, but every day. The sound tech's question – which was basically how to get altered states, enhanced senses, a powerful feeling of belonging to a community and to the cosmos, without drugs – stayed with me, and the seeds were sown for what would become this book.

CONTENTS

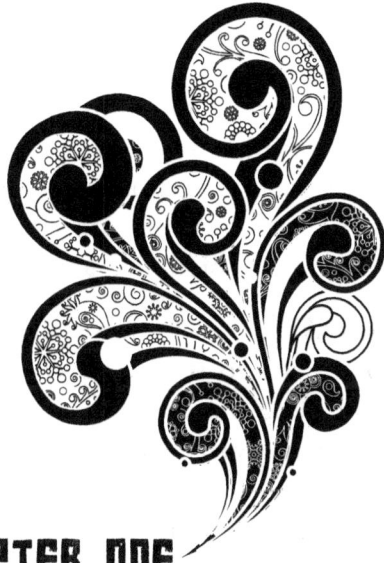

CHAPTER ONE
REWRITING RECOVERY

What did you get right on drugs? It's not the standard first question to clients at a drug recovery clinic. In fact, it's such a radical departure from the standard script that I usually get a blank stare. The recovery industry revolves around the idea of malfunction, but if nothing actually went wrong, that approach doesn't work.

There is a new drug-using demographic – people aged anywhere from 12 to 60, who are rich, poor, old, young, happy, unhappy, male, female, successful, failures, from broken homes or from happy homes – who just like to feel good. With this as a starting point for drug use, it makes sense to look at what went right.

'Revolutionary' is probably the best word to describe this approach, because it does entail overthrowing the old

ost uer

model. And it's old. Most current recovery programs are based on ideas that emerged over a century ago. We no longer ride around in horse-drawn wagons or tap away on typewriters, so why use equally outdated approaches to recovery? It's high time for an overhaul.

Debunking the old myths about why you take drugs is a good place to start. As everyone who has been through counselling or a rehab program knows, identifying 'why' you did it is always the focus. As it is automatically assumed that something must have gone wrong, the answer is inevitably one of the following: you were trying to escape reality, or cope with pain; or you are diseased, self-destructive, have low self-esteem or other psychological problems.

'Drug users are just escaping reality,' is usually stated in an accusatory tone, as if there is something wrong with this. But reality, as most people experience it, is generally so ordinary that, in my opinion, there is something wrong if you *don't* want to escape it. When the police catch runaway prisoners they never say to them, 'Oh, you're just trying to escape prison'. It is expected that you'd flee if you got the chance. But if you take drugs or indulge in any other activity to 'escape reality' everybody gets upset. I believe it is our duty to escape reality and seek an extraordinary life. *How* we do this should be the issue, not *why*.

The idea that drug users are trying to cope with deep-seated pain – usually the 'unhappy childhood' variety – is another flawed assumption. If that was really the cause of addiction, I think there would be many more addicts out there. Growing up can be an unpleasant process, for anyone: you're short, powerless, and your true nature is being systematically suppressed so that you can fit into the accepted limited version of reality. But not everyone takes drugs as a result. Over the years I've treated people for every condition imaginable. Some who adored every moment of their childhoods became heroin addicts. Others who had terrible, abusive childhood experiences never even tried a drug.

Another outdated but still popular theory is that drug users are self-destructive. Well, I spent a couple of decades taking drugs myself, followed by a couple more decades specialising in addiction recovery, and I've never met anyone who started out with a self-destructive intent. No one gets up one day and thinks to themselves, 'Hmmm, what a good day to ruin my life; I think I'll become an addict and an outcast and lie around in gutters'.

More likely, one day a friend or relative offered them marijuana or a pill; they tried it, and then felt even better than usual. Because we live in a world in which drug use is normal and drug imagery and references saturate popular culture, doing it again also seems normal. It is feeling better than normal that kicks off a drug journey. So it is an adventurous and exploratory nature that drives people to repeat drugs, not self-destructive impulses. While the eventual outcome of extensive drug use is definitely destructive, the initial intent is not. This is an important distinction.

It is also commonly accepted that drug users have low self-worth. But these days low self-worth is generally how someone feels *after* doing lots of drugs, not how they feel *before* taking up drugs. The belief that low self-worth is a cause for addiction continues because health professionals are still running on the old script, and because they confuse presenting symptoms with cause. This is an easy mistake to make as, by the time you do seek help for drug issues, you're probably not coming across as a model citizen. You're more likely to be paranoid, twitching and rambling, with the obligatory low opinion of yourself thrown in. If you saw streams of clients in this state, you would naturally assume low self-worth and other psychological problems to be a cause.

Then there is the idea that drug users are diseased. This makes no sense to me. A book I read a while back described how, during the Cultural Revolution in China, Mao had all the addicts rounded up and told that they could either quit drugs or be shot. Needless to say, they all quit on the spot. No problem. In the author's opinion this proved that addiction was not a disease because you could not do that with a group of people who had, say, smallpox. I tend to agree. In my opinion the 'addiction as disease' model is defeatist. It doesn't give you anything to move forward to, whereas looking at what you got right on drugs, does.

It is your duty to escape reality and seek
an extraordinary life

WHY WE REALLY DO DRUGS

There is no great mystery behind why people take drugs; they make you feel good, and everybody likes that. Drugs also reveal the multiple dimensions that make up reality, and I would argue that everybody likes that too. Most of us end up shelving our youthful dreams as part of our induction into ordinary reality, and then resigning ourselves to thinking that life is mundane. One puff on a joint though, and the universe expands, time slows down, every conversation is equally fascinating and hilarious, stress and obligations disappear and eating becomes a sensual feast. You are present and happy, and remember that ordinary reality is not the only option.

Or you might do a line of cocaine or shoot-up or smoke some other speedy-type drug (crack, speed, crystal meth), and get a rush of shattering clarity. A taste of heroin delivers you into a blissful cocoon of forgetting. Or you drop some psychedelic substance or have a nice cup of mushroom tea, and the walls around you melt away to reveal a spinning, luminous universe so beautiful it's beyond comprehension, but you understand it perfectly because you know that you are an integral part of it.

If you felt drawn to repeat a drug experience, you wanted to recapture intense happiness, blissful forgetting or connection to something beyond ordinary reality. You got something very right here, because we are destined to pursue these states. From this perspective, the desire to repeat drugs is not evidence of psychological malfunction or wrongdoing, but rather an indication that you have tapped into something connected to your destiny.

Drug use is connected to destiny

THE RADICAL ROAD TO RECOVERY

Thinking that you got something right on drugs seems counterintuitive, and I would never have dared make such an outrageous claim in my early post-drug days. Like most drug users, I had been brainwashed into believing that drugs are bad, which means that everything you feel and do on drugs is bad and, by default, you are bad.

I would probably have stuck to that script too if I hadn't decided to study Chinese medicine. Although one of the major attractions of study was the opportunity to reinvent myself as a wholesome New-Ager, I found everything about Chinese medicine so fascinating that I threw myself into it with the same dedication I had once applied to scoring drugs. I read everything I could get my hands on, from the ancient books on Chinese medicine to obscure texts on Daoism – the philosophy underpinning traditional Chinese medicine.

I was immediately taken with the Daoists; a group of colourful, eccentric rebels, who sought to live in harmony with nature, crack the cosmic code and escape reality. These were my kind of people. Chinese medicine was my kind of medicine too. The therapeutic platform is neutral.

6

It is based on the belief that organ imbalances contribute to physical and emotional pain and restoring organ function creates health and happiness. There is no 'Let's get to the bottom of your problem' stuff, no making amends and no judgment. Why anyone chose to take a particular path, action or substance is not considered relevant.

After I graduated and accidentally began specialising in addiction recovery, I saw first-hand how this neutral therapeutic approach avoided the emotional traps that delving into 'why' creates. But my clients – mainly people who had become caught in a relapse and rehab cycle – were still concerned with 'why'. They wanted answers. This inspired me to start thinking beyond the commonly accepted reasons. I returned to my study of the Daoist mystics, made the cosmic connection between drugs and destiny, and then everything changed.

*Why you chose to take a particular substance
is not relevant*

FINDING YOUR COSMIC SELF

The Daoists believe that life is meant to be spent as a quest to find the 'cosmic self' and that being in altered states plays a key role in this process. The word 'cosmic' was overused in the hippie era, and for many it still conjures up images of flower children, psychedelic substances and tree hugging. From the Daoist perspective this would be a correct association though, as being cosmic means being more than normal, feeling more than ordinary, and seeing more than 'reality'. This is what the hippies wanted and what every drug user still wants.

While I was thinking about the contemporary application of being cosmic it struck me that it's not actually the drugs you want, it's the way they make you feel. Heightened sensory perception, the expansion of consciousness, overwhelmingly powerful feelings of bonding and love, are all experiences of your cosmic self, so what you really want is access to your cosmic self. Once I made this connection I added 'cosmic' back into my vocabulary, abandoned the idea of neutrality and, scandalously, began working with what drug users got *right*.

A seismic shift occurred. Instead of following the old script – quit drugs or alcohol; engage in a daily battle against powerful urges; finally resign yourself to a half-life spent focused on what you got wrong, and what you will never have again – recovery became an opportunity to recapture heightened states and continue the journey of discovery. 'Find your cosmic self,' became the new recovery goal.

Be more than normal, feel more than ordinary,
and see more than reality

THE CHI FACTOR

Finding your cosmic self is experiential, and achieving altered states again is a part of the recovery plan. This is where chi comes into the picture. Chi is what creates

drug highs. In the West, chi is usually translated as 'energy', but this is too limited a concept. You can get energy from chocolate; you can't get a psychedelic adventure though.

Chi is better defined as being simultaneously energy, information and consciousness. Drugs flood your system with this mix, which is why they can magically convert the dull suburbs into a wonderland, or boredom into thrills. If you want anything in life to feel amazing, trippy or enhanced – just add chi. Chi is the missing link in recovery. If you turn to chi after drugs you can have everything you ever wanted from drugs, and more.

Chi is the medium of traditional Chinese medicine. Treatments such as acupuncture keep your chi flowing. A nutritional diet can build chi. The practices of Tai-chi and Chi-gung can build and move chi but also allow you to download chi. If you learn to work with chi on all these levels you have a recovery lifestyle that heals your physical symptoms and enables you to achieve altered states again. You don't need any fancy equipment, just your body, mind and soul – and chi.

Experience altered states again

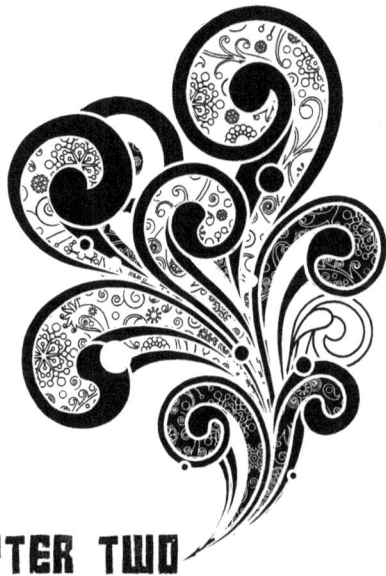

CHAPTER TWO
SOLUTIONS NOT PROBLEMS

Plenty of people will advise you to admit you have a problem so that you can seek help. But admitting you have a problem is part of the old system that focuses on the negative. This creates chi stagnation which, in turn, increases your physical and emotional pain. A positive attitude, however, allows chi to flow. Start thinking about having a solution and all sorts of possibilities appear.

Thinking you have the solution to anything might sound farfetched, particularly in your early post-drug days when you're a gibbering wreck, but if you took drugs to feel confident, socially at ease, happy, creative, empathetic, nurtured, accepting, blissed out and cosmically connected, you have experienced the attributes of your cosmic self. You have a template for what you can achieve again after drugs.

Using a drug past in this way is not such a crazy, or even new, idea. Back in ancient China, some of the mystics deliberately used mind-altering substances to get what they called a 'peak ecstatic experience', to sample their cosmic self. They then sought to recapture what they'd felt without the substances. We have an opportunity to do the same after we quit. Even though the initial intent of contemporary recreational drug use is different, or is assumed to be, all roads can lead to Dao – the fundamental, eternal guiding principle of the cosmos.

As an aside here, although I'm suggesting working with the positives of a drug past by identifying what you got right on drugs, it doesn't mean I'm pro-drug, or anti-drug for that matter. You don't need drugs to experience the altered, enhanced or insightful states that drugs can generate. But if you've already done drugs, I believe you can make that experience into something more valuable than just having had some fun.

> *Don't admit you have a problem, admit*
> *you have a solution*

REWRITE THE PAST

You can revise your past from a solution-based perspective whether you have just stopped drugs or whether it is ten years since you quit. Seeing yourself

purely as having had a problem – or thinking your past was one big mistake – wastes all of those experiences, not to mention the considerable sums of money you invested in mind-altering substances. Value add instead. Rethink your past drug experiences from a new angle and you can convert even the most sordid chapter of a drug past into a potential source of insight.

In the late 1970s, for example, the shine had worn off the drugs for me. I was squatting in derelict buildings in Amsterdam and my only interest was in being high. Each day revolved around scoring and using drugs. For a long time I thought this was just another wasted period (in both senses of the word), but in retrospect, somewhere in there was the seed of something right. Not the part about living desperately in a dingy squat – that's not good for anyone's spirit – but rather that I was prioritising my internal state over all external concerns. All drug users have done this, and if you do it again after you quit, you will have a massive head start on finding your cosmic self and happiness.

Your drug past will hold plenty of material that can assist in creating an extraordinary future. In fact, I now view every part of my progression from nice German boy through pill popper, paranoid dope-smoker, tripper, speed addict, delusional nutter and alcoholic to a depressed chain-smoking suicidal outcast, as having value. Instead of seeing all of that as a waste of time, I understand that I had the right intent – to keep feeling extraordinary – but that it backfired because drugs and other substances are not a sustainable method for achieving this. I went on to find the sustainable method – chi – and my life changed beyond recognition.

Make the switch from drugs to chi and you can forget about problems and instead 'admit you have a solution'.

Get a new perspective on your past

YOU'VE GOT THE POWER

Quit drugs with the radical view that life after drugs doesn't have to be dull, that your symptoms aren't permanent and that everything can change. The more drugs you took, the more challenging it will be to maintain this positive mindset. Especially if you've crossed the line from doing drugs to feel good, to doing drugs so that you don't feel bad, as most dedicated users have. Once the side-effects – stagnation, frustration, irritation, paranoia, fear, panic and madness, to name a few – take over, recreation leaves the building. Addiction and its band of followers, pain, guilt, shame and wrongdoing, enter.

You feel like crap, so it is all too easy to start thinking that everything you did was wrong. But believing this, or that you're bad or that you'll never feel good again, is not useful. You took drugs because you wanted to feel good, and that intent was correct. Wanting to feel good doesn't end when you quit drugs. Given that, spending your time apologising, admitting powerlessness or cleaning toilets in rehab, is counterproductive. It puts you in a position of weakness and you will be more likely to believe the subtexts of 'you did something wrong – naughty you' or 'something went wrong – poor you' which underpin mainstream recovery.

14

Guilt will sabotage your quest to find your cosmic self, as will thinking that addiction is not your fault. Some studies do suggest there is a genetic predisposition towards addiction, but even if this is true, the addiction has to be activated. *You* did that. No one dragged you out night after night and forced you to have a good time (unfortunately). There is always a moment of choice. You chose it, you said 'yes', and you repeated it. You held the power when you did that, so you own everything that happened after that as well.

Don't throw that power away when you quit or you'll fall into the slave class of voiceless, ashamed and powerless ex-drug users. The recreational drugs industry is one of the biggest businesses in the world. I think it's time for the slaves to rise. Join the rebellion, not by trying to change the opinions of others (that's not your job), but by daring to identify some value in what you have done, and then using that knowledge to change your future. We have to fight for success in life in any field, so think 'no surrender' instead of 'I'm powerless'.

Wanting to feel good all the time is correct

SHAME AND APOLOGIES

That's the theory, the application is another matter. Disappointing, betraying, scaring, upsetting, ripping-off or embarrassing those close to you comes with the territory of serious drug use. People have been frustrated, angered, hurt and disappointed by your actions, and reactive cycles have been initiated. These

15

usually keep spinning long after you quit. Some people believe you are a loser who will never change, and regularly share this belief with you. Some may want their TVs back, others want emotional resolution. This fuels shame and reinforces your conditioning to think that drugs are bad and you're bad.

It reinforces the old solution too, which is to admit guilt and make amends. We've all seen those confessional TV shows in which the offending party (drug addict or alcoholic) apologises to the person they have offended (usually the parents or family), then they fall into each other's arms sobbing and, we assume, go home and live happily ever after. But emotional resolution is not usually that simple. We don't see those same people later when the old reactive patterns creep back. Don't get me wrong here; I'm not against apologising. If your desire to do so is genuine, it can be liberating and meaningful for both parties. This isn't the case for the majority of people I treat though, and it wasn't the case for me.

Although I was uncomfortable with the negative effects my drug-fuelled activities had had on some people, there was something about being high that felt so right I could never bring myself to 'admit' that I was wrong. But, because I was physically and emotionally weakened and confused for years after I quit, I also couldn't fight the general consensus that I was a hopeless addict, alcoholic and loser, and that nothing I said, did or thought could possibly have any value. Underneath, though, rebellion brewed. So I reacted. My attitude was that I didn't see why *I* should be the only one apologising when, as far as

I was concerned, everyone else had screwed-up their lives too – just not on drugs. Basically, there was no way I was saying sorry to anyone.

However, I'd always had in the back of my mind that if I ever *was* to apologise to anyone, there was one lady in Nimbin (the infamous Australian drug town where I actually got off hard drugs – only because I couldn't get them there) that I would genuinely be inspired to apologise to. In the early 1980s, while I was at the height of my bizarre post-amphetamine behaviour, she had helped me out with a place to live, immigration paperwork and many other things, and I'd always felt that in return I'd just behaved badly.

Well, I found myself in Nimbin recently, for the first time in many years, and spontaneously looked her up. Even though it was over 30 years since I had left town, she still lived in the same place. We reminisced for a while and then, in a conversational pause, I decided to seize the chance to deliver my apology. I launched into it by saying 'I don't believe in apologies, but ...' She looked slightly bewildered, but I persevered. Turns out she couldn't remember any of the things I'd done. When bits came back to her, like letting her cows into the house or pulling up all her garden plants instead of the weeds, she said, 'Oh you were just a confused kid'.

It was one of those moments where you see yourself or your past actions in a completely different light; maybe I wasn't the total asshole I thought I had been? Anyway, my grand apology scene didn't play out as I had imagined.

Admittedly this was many years later and interior cow herding and scorched-earth gardening were at the mild end of my socially unacceptable activity range. Plus, she was a friend and a drug user herself, rather than a partner or relative. The latter tend to take your imbalanced substance-induced behaviour more personally and are generally not so accepting, and in most cases, with good cause.

Recreational drugs are becoming increasingly potent, and the associated behaviours are becoming more extreme as well. I regularly treat clients who have sold the family home or car for drugs, run amok through the streets, been violent or destructive towards people and property, and then been forcibly restrained and arrested or taken to psychiatric hospitals. Dozens of people may have been involved in these incidents from police to health workers to bystanders. Something more than an apology is needed to counter the scale of the negative aftermath.

Don't get trapped in thinking that drugs are bad and you're bad

MAKING AMENDS

The types of activities that create shame and necessitate apologies are carried out in altered states. You are disassociated from accepted social values. So the solution also lies in altered states and disassociation. Shame doesn't hit you when you are performing sexual acts on your dealer for drugs, stealing from family or friends, selling your body, smashing up bars or committing crimes, because you have either consciously gone through a barrier (and once through, that's it, you can keep going), or you are so out of it you are not aware of your actions.

The shame accumulates though and, after you quit or sober up, memories of your drunken, drugged, shit-talking activities will eventually surface and sabotage your attempts to feel okay about yourself. It might be the next day, it might be years later. Even if you do manage to forget what you've done, those around you probably won't. Apologising doesn't make their memories go away. Time might pass, but the drug elephant remains in the room.

Trying to 'pay your debt to society' by doing good works is not the solution either. I've come across plenty of ex-addicts who became social workers or participated in charitable activities to make amends. This was my motive too for getting into youth welfare work after I quit. I'd been a burden on society and I was going to get a haircut and a job, and do some good for a change by helping young people with their drug and alcohol problems. My new vocation was supposed not only to make up for the trail of destruction I'd left behind me, but also to give my life meaning. It didn't, of course.

All I had to offer back then was the same old 'repent and reform' approach to recovery, which hadn't worked for me, and it didn't work for those I was supposed to be helping. As this became more and more obvious, my post-drug depression and disillusionment grew. My weekends slid into drug or alcohol binges, and eventually I left the profession defeated.

This is a common outcome for many ex-addicts who seek to make amends through charitable actions. A better approach is to be charitable to yourself first, by living in a way that builds your chi and allows access to altered states (disassociation), joy and happiness again.

Make amends creatively

THE COSMIC SOLUTION

In the big cosmic picture, if you generate negative outcomes, whether physical or emotional, a balancing action is called for. Make finding your cosmic self your recovery goal and you will not only neutralise your internal resistance to yourself – which is what shame is – you will have a positive impact on everyone around you. This creates balance.

Lao-tzu, the sixth century BC philosopher reputed to be the founder of Daoism, and the author of one of my favourite books, the *Dao De Ching* – one of the most translated texts ever – said that 'sympathy for others is good, sympathy for self is better'. He got that right. Pursue the cosmic self and you will glow with health and vitality, be fully accepting of everything in your past and be positive in every relationship and interaction. You will also have something other people want. Your presence alone will inspire others to change.

If we ex-users all changed ourselves in this way, it could start a chain reaction of not only personal but also global improvement. The party people would come to the rescue of the planet. What a great way to use a drug past. Everybody wins. This is how you make cosmic amends. As the cosmic version of yourself transforms all your past actions by using them to benefit yourself and others, the triggers for guilt and shame are also defused.

Your recovery goal is to find your cosmic self

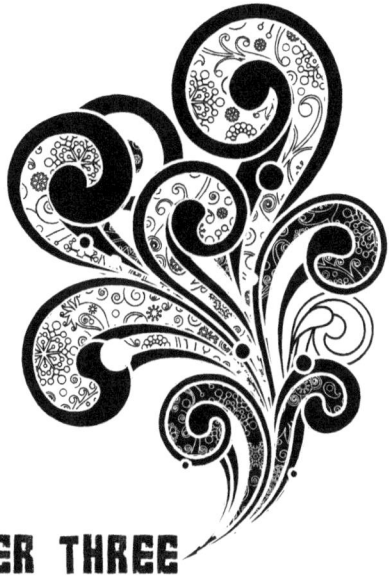

CHAPTER THREE
YIN AND YANG
AND YOU

Addiction recovery is often a long drawn-out process because it gets bogged down in the emotionality of shame, guilt and wrongdoing. Chinese medicine has a refreshingly different approach. From its perspective all actions – even those that we think of as being wrong or shameful – arise from the interplay of the fundamental forces of yin and yang. Yin contracts and yang expands. Yin is stillness and yang is action. Yin and yang balance each other to create harmony. When these forces are imbalanced, disharmony arises. Recreational drug use creates major imbalances.

Everything in the cosmos, including us, is shaped and controlled by these forces. We each have more of a yin or yang type of 'constitution' or fundamental nature. Generally speaking, a person with a yang constitution is extroverted. They have high energy, are quick to engage with people, can forget to eat, get by with very little sleep, have a very high sex drive (the type more likely to initiate affairs), but are also easily aggravated and annoyed. A person with a yin constitution is introverted. They are too shy or selfconscious to engage with people, they can't miss meals, often feel tired, have a lower sex drive and are easily depressed.

Motivational speaker, Anthony Robbins, and real estate tycoon, Donald Trump, are great examples of yang types. Woody Allen, Charlie Chaplin and New Age author, Eckhardt Tolle, are good examples of yin types. Their constitutional types are evident in their actions and also their physiognomy. Anthony Robbins' face is shaped like an inverted triangle with the point at the chin – the movement of energy is upwards and outwards from the jaw. This is a physical characteristic of strong yang types. Robbins is renowned for eating only fruit until lunchtime (only yang types can survive on this diet) and for working incredibly long hours (another yang-type behaviour). Trump, another yang-type man, writes books with titles like *Kick Ass and Succeed* – very yang terminology.

Charlie Chaplin, Woody Allen and Eckhardt Tolle have a different shape to their faces. The movement of energy draws downwards and out, and the base of the triangle would be at the bottom of the face. The way Charlie

Chaplin walked with his feet turned out is a classic yin-type posture; you could push him over in an instant – the opposite of a kick-ass stance. In his movies, Woody Allen often talks about getting a hooker and hand jobs; this is another characteristic yin-type behavior. In excessive yin states you don't have the yang force, or the drive, to maintain an erection long enough for penetration. Eckhardt Tolle famously sat on a park bench thinking for a couple of years. Being able to sit is a yin attribute. Donald Trump would have built a multistory park bench on the spot and then rented the seats out for a profit.

All of the above are highly successful people, because they understand and work with their constitutions. This has a positive impact on every aspect of your life from career choice – different types suit different professions – to relationships. If you are in a relationship with the opposite constitutional type to yourself, it helps to know that nobody is right or wrong in what they do – different sex drives for example – they are simply expressing the yin or yang aspects of their nature. Most of us are somewhere in the middle of the yin and yang range, rather than the exaggerated versions above, but excessive drug or alcohol use can change this.

Drugs reveal something about your true nature

YIN AND YANG AND DRUGS

The effects of recreational drugs can also be described by yin and yang. The speedy substances such as methamphetamine and cocaine are expansive, active yang drugs, whereas heroin and opiates are contracting, passive yin drugs. Even though you may never have heard of yin or yang, as a drug user you have intuitively been working with these forces and your own constitution.

How you planned a party night reveals this, because you probably worked out exactly what to take when to enhance either yin or yang. If you are a high-energy yang-type extrovert, a good night out might have started with marijuana to chill (yin), followed by alcohol to get some action (yang) happening and then, when the alcohol starts slowing you down, some speedy-type drug (yang) to liven things up prior to hitting the clubs again. You might finish off around dawn with marijuana (for a wee dash of yin).

If you are a yin-type introvert your party night definitely doesn't start with marijuana (yin) because this drug will make you too selfconscious to engage, you'll freeze-up (yin) and not make it past the couch (yin) let alone out the door. You might take some methamphetamine or cocaine (yang), to become outgoing and talkative (yang). Then, instead of having a couple of drinks, getting tired and going home, which is what would usually happen with a yin constitution, you can keep on partying with the yang types, but you'll still crash long before them.

Master the forces of yin and yang

YIN AND YANG IMBALANCES

Ongoing drug use creates major energetic imbalances that can bring out the more extreme characteristics of each type. Extreme yang, for example, represents incessant movement. Yang-types who drink heavily and take yang stimulant drugs can become extremely destructive, violent and psychotic. I'm treating huge numbers of crystal meth addicts who party for days and end up making a public spectacle of themselves in psychotic states. Afterwards they are overcome with shame or regret. But their yang urge for movement, their excessive drive, leads them to do it all over again.

This same drive sees them repeatedly going to therapists, and also into recovery and rehab, multiple times. Each time they emerge convinced that they are going to 'change their life, be good, and stay home'. But that yang energy drives them back to their old behaviours and, as their plans to be good never eventuate, they start thinking they are addicts, assholes or diseased. But repeating destructive and aggressive behaviours is not a disease; it is an energetic imbalance. It is an example of excess yang expanding out of control.

Because extreme yin is stillness, yin-type drug users often become depressed and so introverted they are almost unable to move. They don't want to get out of bed, let alone leave the house, and definitely don't want to interact with people. This too is considered antisocial, not normal, so there is something wrong with it. But it is an energetic imbalance. If you forget about right and wrong, shame and guilt, and look at your drug activities in the context of an interaction between your constitutional type and the forces of yin and yang, you've got something practical to work with.

Forget about right and wrong and shame and guilt

YIN AND YANG AND ALCOHOL

The yin and yang model is also perfect to explain many cases of 'alcoholism'. I regularly treat yang success types who believe that they are alcoholics. They have high-stress lives (yang running riot) and then have to drink two or three bottles of wine at night to be able to sleep. Because they need to drink every day, and because they drink alone, they believe that they are diseased. But the real issue is lifestyle and not understanding how to balance yin and yang.

Because these clients have such strong yang constitutions, they get up and get straight into work without food. They might even work through lunch and late into the day without stopping to eat. It's all go, go, go. Again, they do this because their yang energy can sustain them. But there is not enough yin in this equation to allow them to switch over to a yin state in the evening, which is necessary in order to be able to fall asleep. They use alcohol for this.

Instead of focusing on trying to give up alcohol, which goes nowhere, I work with these clients on understanding their constitution and the forces of yin and yang. The goal is to 'evolve' their evening switchover method from bottles of wine to something more sustainable, like potent herbal yin formulas and a chi practice. The latter is great because it teaches how to embrace yang while being in a state of yin. Once they make some lifestyle changes and work with yin and yang and chi, the urgent need for alcohol diminishes and they are able to enjoy a drink socially. I have seen this outcome over and over again. So much for being diseased.

I've treated other 'alcoholic' clients who need excessive amounts of alcohol, usually hard spirits, to get something in their lives that resonates with their yang constitution. I had one client who had been a professional big wave surfer. He loved any sport that had an edge of danger to it (this is an indicator of a yang type). When he retired from surfing, he got a job working as a driver for a sporting goods company. His life became mundane and no longer a match for his constitution. He'd sleep in, skip meals or have snacks and grab takeaway food for dinner. He started drinking a couple of bottles of vodka a night. Initially with friends to re-live the partying, raging adrenalin-fuelled surfing days, but then by himself.

When serious symptoms arose from the alcohol abuse, his doctor told him to stop drinking. But this is not a holistic solution. It doesn't address body, mind and spirit (pun intended). Yang energy needs to move and express itself. This need was not being met in the surfer's lifestyle. I explained all of this, immediately started him on high-powered nutrients and herbal formulas to 'carry' his yang, and also introduced him to Chen style Tai-chi. This is an intense martial art form that resonates with a yang nature. Once he got the idea of working with chi, and yin and yang in the context of his constitution, everything in his life shifted and he no longer needed to get drunk.

Take things up rather than give things up

YIN AND YANG, BALANCE AND BLISS

If you learn how to balance the forces of yin and yang, you can regulate yourself without drugs or alcohol. I treat many addicts who try to suppress their natural drive or yang, because it has led them to trouble. But yang is a gift; it enables us to achieve things.

So, if you are a strong yang type with your yang running out of control, the solution is to work on nurturing yin. This will make you considerate (a yin property). When consideration and drive collide you naturally get a beneficial outcome. Considerate people don't trash bars.

Excessive yin types (and heavy drug use can eventually put everyone in this category) have the opposite problem of being so considerate they are unable to even express an opinion. This is equally debilitating; to be healthy and happy and to find your cosmic self, you need to be able to express yourself freely. In excessive yin states, building yang naturally rectifies the imbalance.

Balance is the secret. The separation of yin and yang leads to pain, but the balance of these forces creates bliss. Ecstasy is a drug that creates the impression of yin and yang in balance, so if you've taken it you know how blissful balance can feel. Working on a great project while under the influence of marijuana is another example of this balance as you are moving forward (yang) and sitting back (yin) at the same time. It's an extremely satisfying feeling. You are sampling 'being while doing', a state highly sought after by the Daoists.

Understanding the interplay of yin and yang is a key to making everything you do after drugs, from sleeping to sex, feel much more satisfying. During sex, for example (and I'm just referring to men here) if you resist that yang excitement and urge for release, instead starting in a surrender mode (a yin mode), when yin and yang come together (pun intended) it can generate chi. Afterwards you'll feel energised and elevated rather than feeling used or ashamed (that old 'morning after the one-night-stand' feeling). Finding your cosmic self is a process that encourages yin and yang to unite, and a blissful life is the eventual outcome.

Balancing yin and yang is a secret to
recovery success

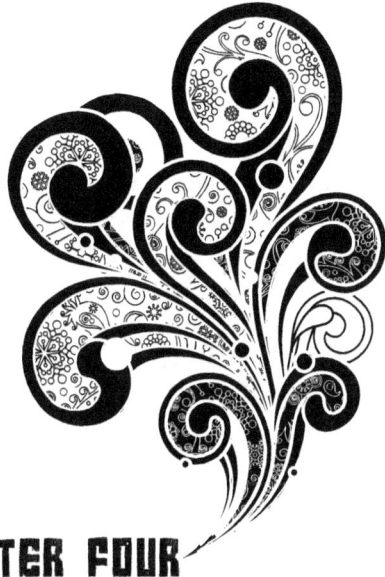

CHAPTER FOUR
REWRITE YOUR FUTURE

The aim of most recovery programs is to take away the substance you abuse and get you back to normal. But taking things away is never the solution. Drugs and alcohol often provide real support for people and this needs to be replaced. As for 'going back to normal', once you've had the experience of being extraordinary, 'normal' is setting the bar way too low.

The Daoists would consider going back to normal as returning to what they call the 'acquired self'. This is the part of your identity that has been constructed by your upbringing, socialisation and the input of peers; it is the self formed by society. It is called 'acquired' because it is something you pick up over time. It is not the real you. The acquired self wants to fit in and be like everyone else. The acquired self feels wounded by the words or actions of others; it seeks revenge; it has judgmental opinions; it criticises politicians; it fights with your partner or kids; and it wants security – oh so badly.

Your cosmic self is the real you. It is accepting of everything and everyone, it has no opinion, it understands the big cosmic picture, it knows that everything you need is within you and that we are all souls on a journey of discovery. The cosmic self knows that we don't come from society, we come from Dao. Being in touch with your cosmic self makes you happy.

We are all destined to experience this and, as drugs give you a sample of this, it's no wonder we like drugs so much, no wonder that recreational drugs are one of the biggest businesses in the world, and no wonder that being high feels so right. It's also no wonder that if you quit drugs and just return to normal (to your acquired self) you'll crave drugs.

Developing an acquired self is something that happens to everyone and partly because we believe that the 'acquired world' or ordinary reality is all there is. But it isn't. Understanding this is critical, because you will lose your place in the acquired world sooner or later. You might be evicted through your drug use, or by the loss of your job, your possessions, your reputation, your health, your relationships or your social status. Or when you join the ranks of the elderly abandoned in retirement homes, or other social outcasts. If you don't know that you have a cosmic option, life can quickly become depressing.

By the time I was 21, I'd been thrown out of college for taking drugs and was living in the underground to avoid the military police who were after me for desertion (German national service) and the local police for, um, other matters. It was only a matter of time until I got hauled off to prison. The speed was no longer delivering extraordinary experiences and, as I thought going back to normal was the only option, I couldn't see a future for myself. I had no idea that I could escape mundane reality, have a purposeful life and continue my cosmic adventures without drugs.

Continue your cosmic adventures without drugs

WE ARE NOT HERE TO BE NORMAL

None of us are here to be normal (acquired). We are here to be extraordinary (cosmic). Escaping reality is our duty. Even though every drug user has had a sample of how this feels, they usually tell me that all they want to do is 'quit drugs and go back to normal'. No one questions this goal, but wanting to go back to normal is like voluntarily returning to captivity after being set free. Imagine the greatest escape movie you've ever seen where, after the wrongly accused and falsely imprisoned hero, who has battled every injustice and obstacle and finally escaped, suddenly decides to get the bus back to prison. It goes against the natural order.

Trying to return to normal after having experienced your true potential is equally unnatural and it will impact negatively on your spirit. It will lead to a separation of yin and yang. If you want to be normal you have to hide your past, because normal people just don't do the sort of stuff you did. Not just the excessive sex and drugs and illicit activities, there's the outright weird too. During the peak of my drug-induced delusion, for example, I took to dressing in robes (which I made myself) and, accompanied by my trusty goat, Schroeder, (yes, really) went on a very public mission to save the world.

I'd like to say Schroeder and I did some good, but I don't think that was the case. Schroeder ended up relocated to a farm. Thinking back, if anyone needed the rural relocation it was me. Schroeder hadn't even done any drugs, he was just slightly confused about his role. I was completely confused about mine.

My messianic visions eventually faded, I put my robes away and may have appeared more normal, but there was no way I'd be discussing my mission with Schroeder at suburban barbeques. It was abnormal behaviour by any standards, as was pretty much everything I'd done since I was a teenager. So I faked normalcy while making sure no one ever found out the truth about me.

Don't return to captivity after experiencing freedom

THE EXTRAORDINARY TRUTH

On drugs you have one life with your substance buddies and another with people who don't do drugs. You don't want to repeat this split personality 'trip' after drugs by pretending to be someone you are not, or pretending your past never happened. Pretense is a characteristic of your acquired self. Pretense stops your chi flowing and encourages yin and yang to separate. Every time that you are not true to yourself you cut off from Dao and feelings of loss, purposelessness or emptiness intensify. Pretense creates pain, which makes you crave drugs.

When you are true to yourself you reconnect, chi flows, yin and yang are more balanced and you feel supported and strong. I discovered this after I became a lecturer in Chinese medicine and realised that I could use my past experiences of addiction, madness and mania to explain the intricacies of Chinese medicine to my students. As most of them had taken plenty of recreational drugs, my unconventional approach to teaching Chinese Medicine proved very popular – until I got fired for not following the curriculum.

I went on to write books and articles adapting ancient Chinese secrets to health and happiness to contemporary life. This led to public lectures and bookshop talks. As heavy drug use accelerates the path to ill health and unhappiness, I started using my crazy drug experiences to illustrate what not to do, and how not to live. It proved an entertaining way to get the message across and I'd often have audiences laughing uproariously. I can confirm that there's nothing quite as liberating or empowering as letting everyone know the truth (as long are you are genuinely OK with the truth). It was then that the emptiness inside me finally started to fill.

By this time I was running my own health centre, so using my past in this way worked for me personally and professionally. If I'd been a bank teller, however, it would have been different. So I'm not suggesting you place ads in the local paper revealing all your deepest darkest secrets and risk freaking out your employers or your granny. It is normal to hide things about yourself that you don't like or think others won't like, but according to the Daoists, we are destined to rebel against social norms that encourage falsity. All ex-users have an opportunity to do this by being true to ourselves, accepting everything we have done and pursuing the cosmic self.

You can't change your past but you can
use it to change your future

ABNORMAL NORMALITY

As drug lifestyles usually begin when you are young, another flaw in 'going back to normal' is that you probably don't know what this means. What most people consider abnormal has been your normal.

Scoffing down my parent's Valium when I was twelve felt normal to me. And everything I did after that – including mushrooms, LSD, mescaline, peyote, heroin, amphetamines, prescription medications, cocaine, marijuana, hashish, opium and various other concoctions – also felt normal. Living in the underground was normal as was smuggling drugs into jail, and dealing drugs. A mohawk and mascara was normal; sleeping during the day and partying all night was normal; taking to the streets with a tennis racquet to hit smoke bombs back at the cops was normal, and driving around with a goat in the passenger seat was normal.

I treat a cross-section of people, but I've yet to see someone who was, say, living a normal life with a spouse and kids in the suburbs, who took up a reckless drug-fuelled party lifestyle during middle age. There probably are drug users like this, because there is every kind of drug user imaginable these days. Anyway, someone like that could have a goal of going back to normal because they know exactly what that means. But for the rest of us, saying you want to be normal is more likely about you no longer wanting to be where you are, physically or emotionally.

Life on drugs might be fun to start with, but at some point it tips into becoming stressful and then gets more so by the day. The side effects creep up on you, and you're always watching out for someone to rip you off or arrest you. You're under financial pressure, as you need much more money than people who don't do drugs, and your physical and emotional pain constantly increases. The stress becomes so unbearable you can end up in the truly abnormal situation where you take drugs to fantasise about being normal.

This is based on a mistaken belief that non-drug-using people live peaceful, pain-free lives (news flash – they don't). This becomes glaringly obvious when you quit, attempt to return to normal and, instead of peace and happiness, you feel emptness and depression. In our culture this is considered a normal post-drug condition. But it doesn't have to be. Rebel against normal expectations.

Don't go back to normal

DON'T LOOK BACK

Going back to normal is an outdated concept. It belongs to a time when rehabilitation meant making you fit back into the acquired world. But we have alternative lifestyles now and I propose adding a new one to the list: 'extraordinary after drugs'. There are certainly enough ex-drug users now (multi-millions and counting) to make this a big movement. Our manifesto will be to recapture the highs.

Let me just say here, that there is nothing wrong with the desire to be normal, and some people may well achieve a return to normal after drugs. I've probably not met them because they're functioning well. The people I treat can't make sense of the normal world, or feel that they don't belong there. Just thinking about another day of ordinary reality makes them want to cry.

If you want to go back to normal, give yourself a couple of months after quitting to rebalance your system and you should be there. But if incessant cravings for drugs and a longing for intensity plague you, and if the only time you feel engaged and inspired is remembering your drug highs, just keep in mind that you can take up the 'extraordinary after drugs' option at any time.

Drugs aren't the problem, mundane reality is

DRUGS AREN'T THE PROBLEM

Everyone promotes the 'return to normal' option because it seems to be the solution to the 'drug problem'. Partners, parents and even kids of drug users regularly come to my clinic seeking assistance to make someone they care about quit drugs. They see the destruction the drugs have created, and naturally think that if you take the drugs away everything (including the drug user) will go back to how it was before.

My clients also fall into the trap of seeing drugs as the problem. They tell me how drugs ruined their lives, their relationships, their career or their future. They blame the drugs; if they hadn't touched drugs everything would have been fine. But seeing drugs as the problem is what led to the 'war on drugs'. This will never solve anything. The problem is not the drugs; it is that millions of us don't find ordinary reality satisfying enough. If we did, we wouldn't take drugs.

The war on drugs was lost before it started, because it targets supply, not demand. The demand is for something more than normal and drugs deliver this. They are a catalyst, a merchant of change; they take you through a doorway to somewhere else. They give you a taste of your cosmic self. If we find new ways of doing this, the war will end and the problem will be solved.

Relying on drugs to keep delivering altered states will create disappointment. I've treated many people in their sixties, who had used drugs for decades and had no intention of ever stopping. They wanted to be able to step out of ordinary reality, or to feel chilled-out or happy on demand. But drugs don't align you with Dao. If you keep using them your chi becomes stagnant, yin and yang separate, negativity and hopelessness rise, you develop an 'us and them' mentality, and lose faith in humanity. Your acquired self dominates. This is the path to misery.

Drugs allow you to sample your cosmic self

QUIT WHILE YOU ARE AHEAD

If you have experienced both your cosmic and acquired selves, you know how much better the cosmic one is. Given this, ideally everyone would quit drugs after one insight into their cosmic self, and then set out to recapture that in an alternative way. This would avoid the painful journey into dark, depressing and acquired territory. I don't know anyone who did drugs once and then quit though. But then again, I wouldn't. I see people who wanted more and more, who were driven to get higher and higher. But if you're on this trajectory, the side effects just get weirder and you become more entangled in the dramas and expectations of the acquired world.

So the next best time to quit is the minute you start noticing side effects. With the speedy drugs, once you get the feeling that your mind is racing ahead of you, quit. Keep going past this point and the suburbs will become populated with spies watching your every move, tapping your phone, bugging your microwave and following you everywhere. You'll need the drugs to hold off the symptoms but you'll eventually lose control over these and your pain and rage will be unleashed. Next thing, you're on a public rampage and it takes a handful of cops to wrestle you to the ground. You're taken away, locked up. There is talk of psychosis, mental illness and medication. This is not very cosmic.

The psychedelics tend to lose their appeal as the trips get darker. I do treat people who keep going regardless though, taking trip after trip until they end up with symptoms including permanently distorted vision, severe paranoia, sexual dysfunction (because they get trapped in overthinking instead of flowing with the desire) or stuck in an unpleasantly altered state. It can be a long way back to cosmic from there.

Opioids, including all those seductive painkillers, which initially create blissful or pain-free states, also take you towards your acquired self. They slowly undermine your core vitality. Once you find you are taking them to maintain normal functioning rather than to surpass it, they are taking you to your acquired self.

Contrary to popular opinion, the old crowd-pleaser, marijuana, also creates side effects. It too takes you away from your cosmic self; it just takes longer to do so than other drugs. If you repeatedly get stoned, imagine or talk about things you want to do, but then never follow though, you're messing with your organ system. Beneath the surface, frustration, negativity and bitterness are slowly increasing. You become cynical about life. This is another attribute of your acquired self; there are no cynical souls.

Aim to recapture the highs

QUIT TO FEEL GOOD NOT TO BE GOOD

As ongoing drug use takes you towards your acquired self, it also encourages the old judgmental (acquired) thinking. This is not only seeing drugs as 'the problem', but thinking that you need to quit because 'drugs are bad'. But drugs are neither good nor bad, they just are.

Quitting because you think drugs are bad, or because you don't want to set a bad example for someone, is the acquired way. But just as we no longer want to live purely within the confines of the acquired world, we don't want to think in that restricted manner either. You took drugs for yourself and although it might sound selfish, you have to quit for yourself. Not because of social pressure, or for your parents, partner, kids, the boss, the neighbours or anyone else. And you have to quit for the same reason you started, which is to do with feeling good.

Don't confuse *being* good with *feeling* good. Quitting because you want to *be* good is acquired thinking. It sets you up nicely for a relapse. You quit, you've 'done the right' thing and 'been good', but then all you get in return is feeling toxic, stagnant and lethargic. You feel ripped-off; you get sick of being good and crave drugs. Or you might think you deserve a reward for being so good, but the only suitable reward you can think of is drugs.

Wanting to feel good doesn't stop
when you quit drugs

EXTRAORDINARY QUITTING

If you quit with an extraordinary intent – not to be good and welcomed back to society (stuff that), but to feel good and find your cosmic self – you'll get an extraordinary result. Remember how you felt when you were high; your spirit soared, you loved everyone, wanted to communicate and bond with fellow humans, and the world was full of boundless possibility? The mechanism for all of that is still there inside you, just waiting for reactivation. If you manage to do that, drug use or addiction can potentially be the most important thing you did.

It was a desire to be more than normal that led you to repeat drugs, and your instincts were right there. So, rebel against the normal recovery script, where everything you did was wrong and you are supposed to forget the past. Everything we do has a purpose. Drugs are here for a purpose and some of us went too far for a purpose. Think about your past from this angle and it will work for you. If you follow the old script and try and forget everything you did, such a great opportunity to discover your cosmic self may not arise again for the rest of your life.

Your Past holds the Key to a Great Future

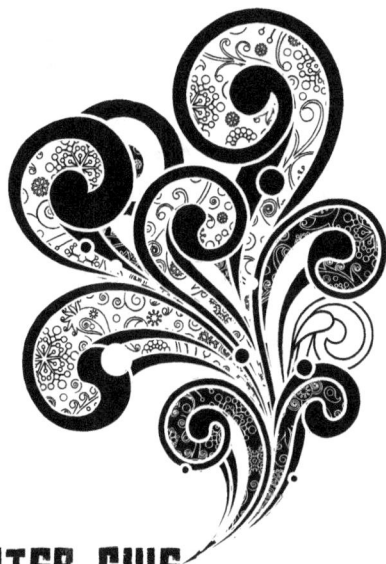

CHAPTER FIVE
EVOLVE YOUR ADDICTION

Rebel against normal expectations by planning to replace one addiction with another. As soon as you quit, cravings will arise. They might manifest as a needle fixation, an insatiable desire for a particular taste in your mouth or the feel of a substance in your bloodstream or just a desperate want for something to take you over. If you direct this longing towards something connected to finding your cosmic self, it can become an asset. The strategy is to 'evolve' your addiction. Otherwise you'll create a liability by turning to non-beneficial replacements such as alcohol, sugar, caffeine or nicotine.

As my speed years came crashing to a halt, emptiness and depression overwhelmed me, so I started drinking. Compared to shooting up speed, drinking was socially acceptable and the hangovers were good for disguising my depression. But, as it turns out, drinking myself unconscious every night proved pretty much as unacceptable as being addicted to drugs. Plus I'd often wake up with no idea where I was or what I'd done.

Once I found myself on a yacht out to sea. I thought I'd been kidnapped (although in retrospect I can't imagine why anyone would want to kidnap a highly inebriated six-foot-four German), but it turns out I'd volunteered myself as crew the night before in some bar. I had no memory of this. What I do still remember though, is that being on a yacht in a large swell is not a good idea when savagely hungover.

Most of my boozy tales weren't so entertaining. I reached the point where I couldn't get through a day without drinking. Eventually I was drinking in parks with other outcasts. Everyone told me I was an alcoholic and had a problem (another one). So I'd buy a full carton of beer but only drink twenty-three cans, leaving one untouched to prove that I could stop if I wanted. Once I realised that the alcohol was just adding to my imbalances, I moved down to the more socially acceptable end of the replacement scale, which meant chain-smoking and endless cups of instant coffee (it was the 1980s).

Prescription medications can become a non-beneficial replacement too. I regularly treat clients who think that medications are 'better for you' than recreational drugs.

But from a Chinese medicine perspective all drugs work the same way: they draw upon your inner resources, your chi, to alleviate pain or change your mood. Your organs can't tell the difference between what we've labelled recreational or pharmaceutical. Medications can further undermine your health and happiness by depleting your chi, and this is why some antidepressants can make you feel even more depressed or even suicidal. Additionally, withdrawal from prescription drugs can be so painful I've seen people get back on recreational drugs just to get off the medications (if you are quitting pharmaceuticals seek professional medical management).

I'm not on an anti-medication rant here. That would be a bit hypocritical coming from someone who enjoyed a wide range of chemical pleasures, including medicinal drugs, for fun. Medications have their place, but becoming addicted to or dependent on them after the recreational drugs is not evolution. You are still on drugs – not to liberate your spirit and feel ecstatic freedom, but rather to dampen urges or suppress pain. This puts you back in mundane acquired territory, and this is not what you signed up for.

Rebel against normal expectations

SEX, DRUGS AND PORN

Shifting from drug addiction to sex addiction is very common. This can be detrimental to health and

happiness, especially for men, as excessive sex drains chi. Sex and drugs go really well together – except for drugs like heroin, which draw chi from your testicles and kidneys to get you high, leaving no energy available for sex – and I treat lots of men who would regularly do three days of nonstop sex and drugs. As both drugs and excessive sex deplete chi, this can create organ imbalances and yang or heat patterns which, in turn, generate conditions such as insatiable desire.

With this type of imbalance you feel an urgent need to have sex but after ejaculation, instead of the post-sex glow, you feel empty, separated or may even find yourself wanting to cry. This prepares the ground for sex addiction because you crave the stimulation of being engaged over and over, to counter the emptiness. But each time you climax, you feel more disconnected. What you are actually seeking here is fulfilment, chi and connection. You're not addicted to sex; you're addicted to chi and connection (we are supposed to be addicted to this).

Internet porn can easily become addictive in a post-drug, chi-depleted situation too. If you are feeling stuck and lethargic, the instant sexual stimulus offered by internet porn (which can set chi in motion) creates the impression of change or movement. But it can also launch a cycle of an increasing need to engage, which simultaneously decreases your inner resources, making the need to engage again more urgent.

I treat sex addiction and internet porn addiction (in clients of both genders) with the same substance I use for drug addiction – chi, because sex and drugs are all about chi. The upside of this is that if you learn to work with chi, you can create states that are like sex and drugs combined. Sex can get better all the time, which improves the quality of life and helps with relationships too.

*There's no limit to how good sex
can be without drugs*

POOR RELATIONS

On the topic of post-drug relationships, it's best to avoid immediately leaping into new relationship after you quit. Because you're feeling lost or empty, it's natural to seek support from others. But in the post-drug weakened state, you are likely to attract an equally emotionally imbalanced person, someone who might be needy, erratic and moody. Everything they say or do will seem wrong and will trigger your anger, grief, or other emotional pain. It's going to be hard to resist expressing this, and endlessly analysing and obsessively finding fault in others. It can quickly trigger major reactive cycles and negativity and cynicism can become a kind of drug replacement.

Or you might be drawn to someone with a really strong character who will be on a mission to change you and get you back to normal. Either way, it will add to your emotional load. So plan for some time on your own, if possible. Don't fall into the trap of thinking that self-worth comes from being in a relationship, because it doesn't. Self-worth comes from healthy organs and strong chi.

Remember that it is your job to fill your own emotional needs, and to evolve.

We are here to resolve ourselves, not others

THE ADDICTIVE PERSONALITY

Many recovery publications and programs propose that there is an addictive personality type, who is likely to replace one addiction with another. Chinese medicine doesn't use this terminology, but if there is such a thing as an addictive personality, you can certainly make it work for you. People often tell me that I have an addictive personality, because I was addicted to drugs, booze, cigarettes, coffee (I became obsessed with tea for a while too) and later, exercise.

There is this theory that it takes 10,000 hours of practice to become brilliant at something. I reckon I did way more than 10,000 hours on drugs, so theoretically I'm really good at being totally out of it. The 10,000 hour theory is usually applied in the context of great musicians, athletes or artists. But you need an addictive, obsessive or driven element in your nature to do 10,000 hours of anything. In the martial arts, they say repetition is 'the mother of skill'. In yoga it is said 'do your practice and all is coming'.

The point I'm making here is that your ability to keep repeating something can be used to your advantage. Of course there are differences between a drug addict and a genius pianist. It is assumed that an addict has lost control, and is no longer making choices, that they *have* to keep repeating their actions, whereas the pianist is disciplined enough to choose to practice for hours every day. That may be true, but in my opinion you can see these as different sides of the same coin. Both are chasing something elusive and something that is connected to an experience of the cosmic self (creativity is another means of experiencing your cosmic self).

Do replace one addiction with another

DEFUSING THE DANGEROUS ATTRACTION

If you direct the obsessive aspect of your nature towards repeating beneficial chi practices, the 'dangerous attraction' of drugs or alcohol disappears. I treat a lot of people who tell me that they have successfully given up drugs or alcohol, are 'clean', and have been for years. But in the next breath, they're telling me how they have to avoid mood- or mind-altering substances, and anywhere these might be available as they are only a step away from falling off the wagon. This is suppression of desire and it leads to a daily battle against powerful urges, a battle which might last you the rest of your life. This is not the front we are supposed to be fighting on.

If you evolve your addiction, the dangerous attraction disappears. You could offer me some of the nicest drugs in town now (and clients regularly do – as a test) and the only thing I would feel is disinterest. I haven't used drugs or smoked cigarettes for decades. Coffee is off the menu too, but only because my overindulgence in that substance once contributed to a seizure. I do like a glass of red wine in the evening, but after one, I'm done; I lose interest in it.

Hard to imagine, since I was supposed to be an alcoholic, and never able to drink again. But my chi practices deliver better highs than anything I ever got from drugs (and in my day the drugs were very good indeed). Anything more than one drink interferes with the quality of the experiences I'm chasing now, so I naturally reject it. I'm not suppressing my desire; I'm fulfilling it elsewhere. I've taken things up a level, evolving from drugs and booze to chi-based altered states. And these I need every day.

Evolve your desires instead of suppressing them

PLAN TO EVOLVE

Thinking about evolving an addiction – like every aspect of figuring out what you got right on drugs – doesn't come naturally. You will need a recovery plan that factors evolution in. Otherwise, you quit while secretly dreading your drugless, aimless, dull future. Then you find yourself sitting in the boring suburbs with no friends – as they are probably drug users and won't want to be with you if you have no drugs – with nothing to do and nothing to look forward to and nothing to think about except how fucking awful you feel, and how much you want drugs. Relapse is inevitable. A plan for quitting and for what comes after that will help to avoid this.

It is generally agreed that there are two recovery stages: acute withdrawal symptoms, for four days to one week, followed by post-acute symptoms, which last from six months to two years. Everyone dreads the acute stage, which is why you tend to quit without thinking the entire process through.

Medical professionals often describe the acute stage as being no worse than the flu. But I'd beg to differ. I've had the flu lots of times and I've quit drugs lots of times too. I ended up repeating the acute stage of withdrawal over and over again. It was like that movie, *Groundhog Day*, but with physical and emotional pain instead of comedy and romance. It was definitely worse than the flu. Additionally, you don't get over the flu and then find you no longer fit in with normal reality.

Then there is the post-acute stage. This is characterised by an inability to concentrate, emotional vulnerability and poor sleep. Somewhere around the two-year mark you are expected to have achieved stability. But insomnia and emotional reactivity were the least of my post-acute stage problems; I wanted to die. It was only the hope that the next day would be different – that I'd wake up and finally be 'back to normal' – that kept me going. I made the mistake of expecting drug recovery to follow the model of normal illnesses or accidents, in which you regain health and wellness and everything goes back to normal. As it became more and more obvious that this was never going to happen, I edged ever nearer to pulling the pin.

Suicidal thoughts are common for a lot of people after they quit, but this is just depleted chi, which means depleted life-force, and it can change. There's really no point bailing out of life early just because you don't know how to quit drugs or, more to the point, how to live after drugs. Plus, pulling the pin while you are operating from your acquired self mode is not a good state to depart in. Dying is a serious business and one that, ideally, we spend our lives preparing for. Making a grand cosmic exit is the plan. Meanwhile we've all got things we are supposed to be getting on with here. So arm yourself with some strategies to build chi and evolve your addiction, and you can avoid a lot of unnecessary physical, emotional and metaphysical pain.

Evolutiononly does one why
Get Addicted to chi

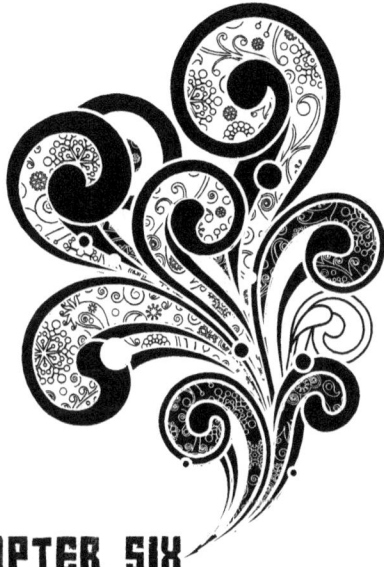

CHAPTER SIX
LOSE YOUR MIND

Evolving an addiction is an experiential process, so you will need to use your body, not your mind. In fact, the Daoists don't ever recommend trying to resolve anything with your mind. We love our minds in the West. Mainstream recovery is based on using our minds to talk ourselves out of taking drugs ('no drugs today, no drugs today'), and then talking endlessly through the post-drug symptoms: the relationship dramas, sexual dysfunction, depression, psychosis, panic and anxiety.

But the mind-based therapeutic techniques were developed by people who didn't spend their time messing with their heads for fun. Once you've done that, your mind is no longer reliable. In Chinese medicine, it's understood that drug use creates a separation of body (yin) and mind (yang), so when you quit, your mind is not anchored. Until you think about taking drugs again, that is, when your mind suddenly focuses on great ideas like 'maybe do drugs one more time, then you can quit', or it starts hammering on about what a loser you are, or setting off endless debates about right and wrong.

Clients regularly tell me that they hate their thoughts but can't escape them. This is the situation in which your mind can be described as 'the enemy of Dao', because it is sabotaging your health and happiness. Once it enters this enemy territory, you will automatically be putting a value on your own or others' actions. You become opinionated and judgmental and you move further from your cosmic self. From this perspective, the old approach to recovery – in which you consciously focus on wrongdoing, and are expected to make value judgments on your past – can be counterproductive.

Don't try and resolve the past

SENSE THERAPY

Drug use does take you into pretty dark territory and activities that are considered shocking by normal standards. When you talk to anyone about these, it immediately engages their senses. If their senses then direct their thoughts, they will feel disturbed or disgusted and they will put a value on your actions based on socially accepted ideas of right and wrong. Then the probing begins; they need to know why you did it or what went wrong to make you do it. This can go in circles for years without resolution. It's a mind trap.

The Daoist alternative is to learn how to direct your mind to chi instead of to senses. Chi is always empty, so the moment you turn to chi you are empty. In emptiness, whatever is, is. The universal truths are revealed. Being able to direct your mind to chi creates a state called 'choiceless awareness'. A therapist who can access this state won't be sitting behind their desk looking carefully expressionless while secretly thinking 'oh my, this person has really screwed-up, really done some bad things, tut tut'; a drug user won't be forever judging their past actions in light of what they got wrong, and then getting mired in shame and guilt.

But you can't experience choiceless awareness without a dedicated chi practice. I do four hours chi practice each day, so that when treating a client, I can instinctively go into a state of chi. Then I don't see an addict, a depressive, a psychotic, an obsessive; I see another soul. Imagine what the world would be like if we all could all see each other like this all the time.

This is not to say that there is no place for talk therapy; your mind definitely does have a role to play in recovery. I always start my treatments with my signature shock tactic consultation, where I get the person to rethink their substance use. Seeing the positive in your past makes chi flow. But I follow the consultation with a specific acupuncture treatment, which creates an altered state and brings the body into the equation as well. So you see things differently in your mind – chi flows – and then you feel things differently in your body – chi flows. This is an approach to therapy that keeps you on the cosmic path.

See the positive in your past and
your chi will flow

BRING YOUR MIND BACK HOME

In Chinese medicine psychology is in the body, not the mind. So your recovery strategy is to 'lose the mind' and turn to the body. This will naturally bring your mind back home. Now, when I say 'body', I'm actually talking about your organs. They house your mind. This might sound outlandish, but if you were happy with ordinary explanations about life, you wouldn't have repeated drugs.

The mind and mental activities – intention, will and thought – are governed by your organs (your spleen plays a major role in this). The spiritual gurus consider the mental functions to be a divine gift. High on a drug like ice you can see why because, as that drug really enhances spleen function, you temporarily experience intention, will and thought perfectly harmonised. There is no gap between planning and action. Whatever you decide to do happens immediately and effortlessly. Ultimately, this is how we want to be operating all of the time and, given that this is reliant on building organ function and chi, we can.

If you've done a lot of speedy drugs though, it can be a long way back to this place. Those drugs take a toll on your organs, particularly your spleen, and the relationship between intention, will and thought fractures. This is how you 'lose the mind', in the negative sense. Instead of providing focus and clarity, your spleen – which is also the drama queen of the organs – freaks out, and you feel scattered and consumed by jealousy, yearning, resentment, procrastination and worry. You are confused about who you are and what you are doing here. Paranoid scenarios loop in your head about who said or did what to you. Your actions no longer make sense.

A classic example from my past: one morning at work after a three-day speed bender (while I was working as a drug and alcohol counsellor), I had to photocopy some documents. I decided I needed a coffee before facing the task, but in my scattered state I spooned coffee and sugar onto the photocopier instead of into a cup. I immediately panicked and fumbled around frantically trying to clean it up before anyone realised how mad I was. In hindsight I should have first pressed the 'copy' button to get a memento of what happens when you have trashed your spleen and ended up with no connection between intention, will and thought, because that's what was actually going on there.

At the time I feared for my sanity, and that's a terrifying feeling. I regularly treat people who have taken so many drugs that they are no longer capable of normal communication. They might think in symbols or speak in jumbled words, or streams of consciousness. Whereas Western medicine identifies this as mental illness, and treats it with more drugs – which further separate body and mind – Chinese medicine addresses the underlying organ imbalances. Your mind comes back home and regains optimum function. It becomes a powerful asset in the search for the cosmic self.

Make your mind work for you,
not against you

PLAYING THE ORGANS

The organ model not only logically explains weird drug-related symptoms and states, but also the much debated 'gateway cycle'. Although I had progressed from marijuana to hard drugs myself, I never bought into the gateway theory until I studied Chinese medicine.

I turned to speed because marijuana (and hashish) had stopped working for me. But plenty of people around me happily continued smoking dope, thus debunking the gateway cycle myth, or so I thought.

In fact, this was due to the interaction of their constitution and yin and yang, but I didn't know that then. All I knew was that marijuana might have failed me, but one line of that magic white powder and I was back. I was instantly up, out of the beanbag, making speeches and planning to take over the world. Unbeknown to me, the paranoia and lethargy I felt were the result of marijuana's yin effect on my liver. The speedy drugs corrected this, as they brought the qualities of the spleen into the picture. But as the amphetamines wreaked havoc on my spleen I began to seriously lose the plot.

The next step in the gateway cycle is heroin, which impacts on your kidneys. These are known as the 'mother of yin and yang'. They house your willpower and your life force. Powerful kidney energies can temporarily override spleen dysfunction and make the speed-induced emotional pain and confusion disappear. Heroin is the last stop in the gateway cycle though, because it taps into the very source of your power reserves. This is why the side effects are accelerated ageing – obvious in the skin, teeth and organs – but also increasing fear and loss of willpower.

There is a gateway cycle, but it doesn't end with heroin, you can keep going with chi. This is the ultimate mood- and mind-altering substance. You probably won't have heard the gateway cycle, or the mind, drugs or recovery for that matter, explained from this perspective before, but it makes sense.

It explains why and how you feel so bad when you quit. If your organs are depleted your lungs generate grief; your liver, frustration; your spleen, confusion; your kidneys, fear; and your heart, depression. No wonder you feel purposeless, disconnected, lost and mad.

But the organ model also offers a path forward. Evolve your addiction via a chi-building lifestyle that improves the physical and metaphysical function of all your organs, and your lungs will generate spontaneity; your liver, happiness; your spleen, boundaries; your kidneys, power; and your heart, love. No drugs required.

Keep the gateway cycle going all the way to chi

FOLLOW YOUR FEELINGS

You became an addict or committed drug user because you followed feelings, not theories. Take an experiential approach to recovery and engage directly with your feelings again. If you are still using drugs, you can get this process underway before you even quit. I regularly develop plans for clients where there is an overlap period in which they might still be engaging with the old drug lifestyle, but at the same getting treatments and making lifestyle changes that establish a new rewarding lifestyle.

This way, right from the start the emphasis is on replacement and feeling good, and you can avoid wasting time getting bogged down in theories about where everything went wrong. I've read a lot of recovery books written by addiction professionals who have never taken drugs. And while these may have helped many people, for me, it's like reading a cookbook written by someone who has never eaten food. The altered states, the magic and the mystery are missing. Chi delivers these and it's not theoretical. This is why we need to focus on the body.

Even if drugs could keep delivering, the experience eventually becomes 'so what'; you become cynical about the highs. Do drugs for ten years and I can guarantee you're going to feel like crap. Do chi practices for ten years, though, and you're going to feel awesome. You can keep reaching higher and more intense states.

Quit to feel good, not to be good

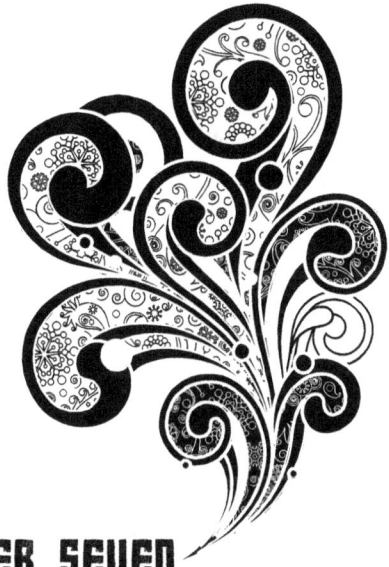

CHAPTER SEVEN
QUIT WITH YOUR BODY

There are three practical components to quitting with your body: correct deficiencies, repair the damage and then align. Tackling deficiencies and repairing damage comes first. This replenishes your chi reserves and improves organ function. I immediately put clients on high-powered nutritional supplements and herbs, introduce a nutritious diet, get them started on some form of exercise and start regular acupuncture treatments.

Nutrient deficiencies are one of the major reasons you feel like crap after quitting and the best way to get nutrients back in as fast as possible is nutritional supplements. These are concentrated high-quality food. They can build chi, help break down energetic blockages and correct the imbalances that drug use created. They assist your life-force to come forward again so you are motivated to move. I've been researching nutrient therapy in relation to addiction for decades now. I studied, and then lectured in orthomolecular therapy, which works with high doses of vitamins (such as vitamin C for addiction) but I've since investigated the properties of not only nutritional supplements but also the superfoods, which are undergoing a major revival.

Every plant on earth has a unique property. Drug users are obviously very familiar with this concept (think marijuana, the poppy or the magic mushroom) but this applies to every plant from ginseng to peas. Plants can't escape their environment so they develop a specific 'adaptive' intelligence. For example, acai berries, which grow right at the top of palm trees under the blazing equatorial sun, are cool inside when they are picked. This is nothing short of astonishing; we'd fry in about two minutes up there. Acai has a highly developed antioxidant function, and when we consume acai we can benefit from that.

Chinese herbal medicine has long recognised and worked with the concept of plant intelligence. There are herbal formulas to correct specific organ imbalances, build physical and emotional strength, and to support the seeker of altered states. If you draw upon both Eastern and Western nutrient knowledge you can create a transformative powerhouse of supplements and superfoods that will alleviate withdrawals and cravings, accelerate the healing of post-drug symptoms, and assist in rebuilding the high level of organ function needed to naturally achieve altered states again.

Many people resist the idea of taking nutritional supplements. I can't count how many times I've heard people claim that if you have a healthy diet you don't need vitamins or supplements. This is simply not true. Maybe it was in our distant caveman past when there were no vitamin companies and we ate hairy mammoth off the bone, but these days food is more likely to be entertainment than nourishment. Most of what we eat is so processed and the sugar content so high, it actually depletes your life-force.

Even a purely organic diet is not enough to keep anyone healthy in our culture, let alone rebuild someone who has had a depleting drug lifestyle. So get into the supplements. Working with the power of plants to make yourself feel good is second nature to you, so continue this with a different range of feel-good plants. Nutrient therapy is a complex field though, so seek professional input.

Work with the power of plants

FOOD AND CHI

Food is a source of chi and you can use meals to regulate your moods, the same way you once used drugs. Every meal you eat should make you feel grounded, calm and energised. You need warm, wholesome cooked meals for this. A general example of a grounding, chi-building menu would be porridge for breakfast; meat, vegetables and rice for lunch; and either rice and vegetables or soups in the evening. Avoid highly processed entertainment foods. They deplete chi and block chi flow, which leaves you feeling ungrounded, aggravated and tired which, in turn, creates cravings.

Drugs take a toll on your digestive functions, so this menu might be a bit ambitious, especially immediately after quitting, when you're probably no longer used to eating regularly, and you are likely to have food intolerances (from organ deficiencies). Start with soups and stews, and work your way up to more substantial meals.

This is not the time to become a vegetarian. You need nutrients and protein to build your organ function. Otherwise the likelihood of depression, unpleasant head spinning and other ungrounded sensations will increase and you'll want drugs to make these feelings go away.

I accidentally became a vegetarian when I arrived in Nimbin in the early eighties, as hippies didn't eat meat. I'd been doing speed daily for a long time by then; my spleen function was seriously impaired and I was already scattered and weird. Luckily, most of the locals were in a similar state, not to the same extent as me, but enough to make me blend in. I lived in a commune in the hills with extreme alternative types. Everyone grew vegetables and, being flat broke, I ate pumpkin at least three times a day.

Pumpkin is actually good for your spleen, but deprived of protein I had the drug parrot on my shoulder the whole time whispering in my ear. It didn't want any more pumpkin; it wanted to party. Twelve months later I took a job as a ski instructor in a mountain town and hit the powder, in more ways than one. I started shooting up speed again. My spleen and other organ functions plummeted, reality eluded me and shortly after that, Schroeder and I took to the road on our mission.

If being carnivorous is simply not an option, make sure you get a really good alternative source of protein. Avoid crazy detox diets too. I've treated plenty of people who quit drugs and then turned to raw food or juice fasts to 'cleanse' or 'detox' themselves. Yes, you will have a build-up of toxins in your body, so it is normal to feel contaminated or dirty after quitting, but detox diets can create a toxic overload that ultimately makes you feel worse. Raw foods can take more energy or chi to process than cooked foods, and after drugs you need to be nice to your organs and nurture and build chi. Wholesome cooked food, nutrients and herbal detox formulas are a better option.

Use food to regulate your moods

EXERCISE AND CHI

Your body is the interface between your mind and the external world, and you will be feeling physically uncomfortable after you quit. This makes communication difficult, increases your emotional pain and creates the desire to withdraw. Exercising can quickly change this by generating physical fluidity, helping get your mind back into your body and creating feelings of wellness. In some countries, exercise rather than antidepressants is now prescribed as the first treatment option for depression.

I discovered the power of exercise firsthand while I was working in social welfare and desperately trying to hide my post-drug depression. I'd hooked up with a new sporty girlfriend and we'd gone to a pool for a swim (her suggestion, not mine). I started enthusiastically doing laps to encourage her to see me as a normal person who did normal things, like swimming, as opposed to shooting up drugs in a squat somewhere. But to my surprise when I got out of the pool I actually felt good. By then I'd completely forgotten that you could do so without drugs. That was the moment I turned into a weight-lifting, swimming, running, cycling, gym-junkie. If I could have exercised while I was asleep, I would have done.

Hardcore exercise is critical for those who've done the heavy drugs such as speed and ice, as they create massive chi stagnation and an overload of toxins. You need intense workouts to help push this through your system. It's common to have reduced muscle tone and increased body fat after drugs too, and a strong weights/cardio program can get this ratio back in balance so that your organs can breathe and your chi can flow again and re-energise you.

I'm big on maximising the benefits of everything you do, and I always suggest adding therapeutic value to exercise. For example, if you are doing squats and treadmill or stationary bike work, as your muscles burn, you can visualise burning negative thoughts and replacing them with positive ones. Repetition of this process helps to hardwire positivity as your default state. So when negative thoughts, images or ideas come up, as they regularly will in the emotional minefield of life after drugs, it is much easier to replace them with positive ones.

Use exercise to create feelings of wellness

THE ENDORPHIN RUN

Exercise is definitely an important part of feeling extraordinary after drugs but on its own, it's not enough. I regularly treat people who quit drugs, go to the gym every day and exercise hard but still relapse. There's something missing and it's not endorphins. Parents of young drug users often ask me, 'Why can't they just go for a run instead to feel good?' But, as I explain to them, for most drug users, pounding the pavement in agony with burning muscles while gasping for breath, in the slim hope of an endorphin release – a piss-weak cousin of any drug high – is not a satisfactory replacement.

Even if it was, you can't run all day every day, and what happens if you break an ankle or the weather turns nasty for a couple of months? Or if you live in one of those cities where you only run if someone's chasing you? Don't get me wrong here, running is a great thing to do (if you can) not only for physical strength, but also for the satisfaction of breaking through the post-drug inertia and feeling back in control and, of course, there's no point knocking back an endorphin rush. But my theory on running and exercise in general is that it is part of ordinary reality; you're still 'here'. It's not a multidimensional experience. If you want to fully replace what drugs delivered, you have to go into the mystical territory of chi.

Don't settle for endorphin highs

CHI TREATMENTS

If you are in perfect health, chi flows throughout your body. It nurtures your skin, tendons and muscles, so you can move smoothly and effortlessly (as you would dancing on ecstasy), and it also flushes through your internal organs, allowing optimum physical and metaphysical function. You feel awesome, you love everyone and everything, are connected to all there is, and your life feels purposeful.

Drugs force chi to rush along your meridians – an invisible network of chi pathways in your body – which is how they create these great states, but drugs simultaneously deplete your reserves of chi and cause obstructions to build up at the acupuncture points. Eventually these points become so blocked that chi can't move freely, so your body aches and you feel physical and emotional pain. When acupuncture needles are inserted at these blocked points the obstruction is instantly reduced, chi can flow and you feel good again.

But we want more than good, we want extraordinary. In Chinese medicine, the cosmos is seen as a massive chi matrix. Acupuncture not only allows chi to flow internally through your body, but externally to and from the matrix, too. Some acupuncture points are actually 'vortex' points that open up to other dimensions. Because chi is energy, consciousness and information, the acupuncture needle can act as an antenna that can access cosmic information and chi. It can be a totally psychedelic modality.

Each of your organs (we have twelve organs in Chinese medicine, including an invisible one, which is pretty interesting) has a spark of cosmic consciousness. I have developed a specific form of addiction recovery acupuncture that can temporarily create a state of internal organ function high enough to reignite that spark. This accelerates physical and metaphysical healing.

So, for all these reasons, getting daily acupuncture treatments as soon as you quit (or beforehand), is highly recommended. Then shift to weekly treatments. Don't start thinking that you're cured once you feel some improvement. Drugs create massive chi stagnation and imbalances, and the more drugs you did, the more treatment you will need and the more time it will take to recover. But also, unlike Western medicine, where you see a doctor when you get sick and then take a medication to make your symptoms disappear (usually they just go somewhere else), Chinese medicine aims to heal underlying imbalances. If you commit to regular treatments you will be starting a trajectory of limitless improvement.

Chinese medicine supports you on the path to your destiny

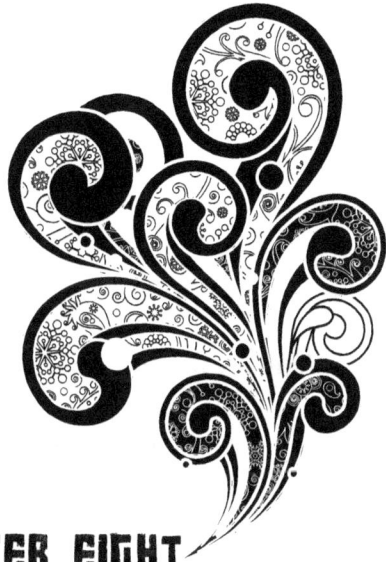

CHAPTER EIGHT
THE POWER OF CHI

Taking up yoga, Chi-gung, Tai-chi or another martial art is a critical part of your recovery plan. These practices involve moving through a series of postures that allow chi ('prana' in yoga), to flow around your body. The techniques were created centuries, if not millennia, ago on top of remote mountains or deep in distant jungles by outcasts and misfits who were not interested in having a boring or normal life (sound familiar?). The chi practices build health, but they are also the means to escape reality.

An increasing number of mainstream rehab centres have begun offering yoga or Tai-chi, seeing them as nice calming or stretching exercises. And they are, but that's just the start of it. The Chinese chi practices (Tai-chi, Chi-gung) were developed after centuries of observation of extraordinary animal abilities The practices copy these skills and allow us to escape our perceptions of physical limitations. Jackie Chan's famous gravity-defying movie stunts are a great example of this. But this is just the start of where chi can take you.

If I'd had any idea of the trippy origins and real power of these practices, and the states they can put you in, I would never have done drugs, I would have apprenticed myself to some Tai-chi master or guru instead. But I'd never even heard of chi when I had my first joint, and I followed the drug path to altered states instead. Things are different now. We might be experiencing one of the biggest recreational drug epidemics in history, but simultaneously, and for the first time ever, amazing once-secret chi techniques are now widely accessible. The internet is saturated with footage of great martial arts masters demonstrating superhuman capabilities. It's never been easier to go from drugs to chi (or to skip drugs and go straight to chi). So turn to chi right now, right away.

Chi allows you to escape reality

HARD DRUGS AND INTENSE CHI

If you've been a hard drug user, you will have major imbalances of yin and yang. You may well have a condition known as 'yang rising', where all your energy is up in your head, creating an empty, heated intensely

irritating sensation. When you take up a chi practice you need to keep a few things in mind. For example, if you are learning Tai-chi or Chi-gung, teachers will instruct you to 'relax' but you are probably physically unable to relax, so you'll feel frustrated and start thinking chi is not for you. Think 'sink in, sink in' instead of 'relax' and it will work better for you.

You can adapt a lot of what you have instinctively learned about chi from your hard drug experiences. For example, you feel a drug rush start in your belly because it is activating the primal energies in the body. This is the Dantian, the seat of power. This is where you 'gather' chi.

When I teach Chi-gung, I begin by putting the client in the basic standing posture – feet hip-width apart, knees slightly bent and spine upright – and then get them to place their hands on the lower belly. The Dantian is where you start to reconnect with chi again after drugs. Your familiarity with moving a drug rush internally is also something that can now be applied, as the next step is 'directing' chi.

If you took a lot of hard drugs I'd recommend learning intense martial arts forms as well, because you'll need something powerful to counter the pull of these drugs. I regularly treat people who tell me that after they quit, the darkness keeps calling them back and they just want to give in to it, and go back to jail and so on. Martial chi techniques are essential to engage with the darkness, to merge yin and yang, and to liberate yourself from the memories that constantly return you to dark actions.

If you are drawn to the dark side, go as hard on the chi as you did on drugs. Take up Chen-style Tai-chi (my favourite) or Praying Mantis Kung Fu, which has a vicious aspect that can meet the intensity of that darkness and enable you to transform it. If that feeling of being drawn to the darkness becomes overpowering, I'd do a couple of hours hard chi work in the morning and another less intense hour in the evening. No days off, no discussions, no contemplating. Just do it. Otherwise your life can quickly become hell.

You need a teacher and a school for any chi practice. If you can't find a teacher right away try video tutorials, books or DVDs, but getting a teacher is best. Get into it as soon as possible and immediately start practising every morning. Ideally, outside and near trees as you can pick up more chi (hugging trees on LSD makes sense from this perspective). Even if you barely know what you are doing and feel like a fool, just keep doing it (the practice that is, not the tree-hugging). You'll get more and more insight into where chi can take you. Repetition also builds the emotional strength and willpower necessary to stay on the extraordinary path. Plus, quitting drugs with a technique that enables you to feel good and to escape mundane reality is a no-brainer.

Chi can counter the attraction of drugs

RETURNING TO CENTRE

You can use a chi practice to return yourself to centre too, when you feel you are about to lose it, or if your mind starts racing with that manic psychotic energy

(yang rising). Instead of engaging with the triggers, turn to your body (yin).

Step away, go outside (or anywhere) and do some slow squats. Slowly sink down, exhaling, and thinking 'trust'. Then slowly rise up, inhaling, thinking 'acceptance'. Keep the focus on the Dantian, your power centre, and send your awareness to your legs. Breathe into the muscles in your calves and thighs. Repeat until you feel centred again. This is a simple strategy, but it builds yin, which is a natural antidote to the yang states of panic, anxiety and delusion, so it will quickly create emotional stability.

Being highly susceptible to anxiety and panic is normal after drugs, but if you do your chi practice daily, you will be constantly balancing yin and yang, so these body/mind imbalances won't get on top of you. If you drift away from the practice though, they can quickly come back. Many years after I quit drugs, I'd get recurring anxiety attacks. They were always connected to stressful times in business, and disrespecting yin. During one of these periods, I had to fly on a business trip to Asia. I started getting anxious about the prospect of being in a confined space up in the air with no escape, and I started panicking about it.

Panicking about panic was just getting ridiculous, so I made an appointment with a psychologist. I hadn't done that before. Once you've been on a mission with a goat, you tend to avoid those who examine your sanity as a profession. But the therapist part of me is always interested in other therapeutic approaches, and there was really no need to mention Schroeder (I hadn't seen him in years), so off I went. They told me there was no biological basis for panic attacks and, as I didn't want medication, they suggested I try mindfulness techniques. The idea was to focus on being in the present and to sit with the emotion rather than reacting to it.

Basically the strategy was to use thought to conquer thought. It was all very rational. But you can't hold rational states with major organ deficiencies and yin and yang imbalances. Thought is already unable to control thought or you wouldn't be panicking. So it was unsuccessful for me. I did board the plane, but struggled with waves of anxiety and panic for the next ten hours. By the time we landed I was sweating, twitching, and looking more like a drug smuggler than when I actually had been one. I was fully expecting to be arrested and executed.

I had forgotten the incredible power of yin. I'd fallen into the yang success trap of thinking I had to do 'whatever it took' to achieve my goals. I had temporarily stopped doing Tai-chi, thinking it was too 'slow'. This is the road to failure, not success. Being so yang created imbalances, and anxiety and panic resulted. As soon as I got back into the chi practices my symptoms receded.

Anxiety has nothing to do with the mental processes, so you can't resolve it with your mind. Metaphysically, anxiety attacks are 'fire' out of control. Your internal balance has been so disrupted that the fire that is supposed to be fuelling your destiny is raging in the wrong direction. You correct this through your body.

Chi can alleviate panic and anxiety

RESOLVING TRAUMA WITH CHI

Another good reason to take up a chi practice, if you don't have enough already, is its therapeutic benefit. You can eventually build such emotional and metaphysical strength that you can look your most painful memories in the eye, both the things people did to you and the things you did to other people, and think 'so what'.

According to Chinese medicine, traumas are stored in your body in the form of toxic energy. Drugs suppress this, but when you quit it will come forward. Your life might suddenly seem to turn to crap, and you feel as if 'trouble follows you' (I hear this all the time from clients). If you don't understand why this is happening it is very tempting to go back to drugs to handle it. But this will just make everything worse.

Despite what I said earlier about unhappy childhoods and addiction not necessarily being connected, I do treat people who became addicted as a result of self-medicating for emotional or physical trauma, usually experienced in their early years (it's just not the majority of drug users who start this way). It's not unusual for me to see people in their thirties or forties who may have only had seven or eight non-medicated years; usually their first seven or eight years of life.

Plenty of people have terrible experiences in their childhood, but they don't take drugs. They might suppress these memories or develop some other coping mechanism, but they are still 'here' in ordinary reality. If you used recreational drugs to self-medicate for pain and trauma, you have chosen a different option. Talk and mind therapies work within the framework of being here, but your recovery has to include a method to process trauma within the framework of disassociation, of being 'elsewhere'.

Chi practice puts you into an altered state; it takes you into the realm of 'elsewhere'. The chi postures clear blockages in the pathways in the body where the toxic energy of past traumas is stored – mainly the thighs, legs and lower back – allowing it to release. It's no coincidence that activating these muscle groups is a core component of both Tai-chi and yoga. The idea is to tune into the painful memories or feelings as you do your practice and you will slowly release and transform them.

So, if sitting on a therapist's couch feeling like a loser or sobbing as you revisit every terrible incident from your past, isn't your style of therapy, or you can't face doing this yet, the chi practices are a great alternative. People spent thousands of years working these systems out and they are extremely effective. I have been doing chi practices daily for more than thirty years now and I can't emphasise enough the power of chi to change everything – to resolve painful memories and to heal.

Even if you didn't start using drugs to deal with pain, recreational drugs often end up being used for this purpose as, regardless of how happy and cheery you were when you began, once your intake reaches a certain level you are creating major imbalances. At some point you switch from using drugs for fun to using them to suppress symptoms. This pain will be stored as toxic energy in your body and when you quit, it will come forward.

The path after drugs is the liberation of the soul, the processing of trauma or karma, the merging of yin and yang. So make chi your priority and your lifestyle becomes an ongoing therapy, processing not only your past but also the ongoing physical, emotional or spiritual hurdles that are a natural part of life on this interesting planet.

Chi can process your pain

DAILY CHI MEETINGS

Finding your cosmic self after drugs is not an easy path. All the gurus, yogis and Daoist masters knew this. This is why they developed chi practices. Do a chi practice every day, otherwise you'll feel like you are on your own and the desire to relapse into your old negative or destructive behaviours may be overwhelming. The chi practice makes you feel supported and connected to yourself, to other people and to your soul family.

You want your chi practice to be playing the role of a friend. This might sound weird, but if you're a committed user, drugs probably felt as if they were your friend. Try to recapture that relationship with chi. None of us are here to go it alone. We are supposed to see and feel the path ahead, and feel supported as we follow it. The chi practice will do this and connect you to Dao. So learn the arts and fight to stay on the path to a future of ecstatic freedom. Do it now and don't ever look back.

You were addicted to chi, not to drugs

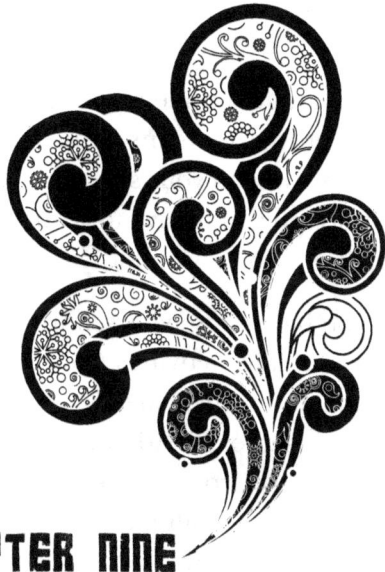

CHAPTER NINE
GO WITH THE COSMIC FLOW

Chi is the medium to find your cosmic self. It is limitless and the more you work with chi, the more extraordinary your life after drugs will become. The idea is to make everything revolve around chi, the way it once revolved around substances. You can build chi and move chi, but you can also conserve chi and even download it from the cosmos.

Chi is everywhere and it flows through everything in the universe, including us, in a twenty-four hour rhythm. It is as regular as clockwork. This is known as the chi cycle. If you had one of those red laser dots tracing the movement of chi through your body it would move to your lungs at

3 am and continue working its way around, visiting each of your twelve organs in turn. In fact, if you could see that dot moving on your skin you could throw your watch away (although you'd have to strip whenever you needed to tell the time, so maybe not).

If you harmonise yourself with this flow, by doing all your normal daily activities (eating, sleeping, having sex, etc.) at the times when specific organs are energised, you build and conserve chi. Add in chi practices at certain times and you also set yourself up to be able to access cosmic chi. This is what I call a chi-cycle lifestyle, and it's my 'secret recovery weapon'.

Technically, of course, it is not actually a secret. Centuries ago, after spending a very long time closely observing how the universe functioned, the Daoists not only discovered chi, but also realised that chi flows in this cycle. They worked out how to align their lives with this to maximise health and happiness.

Applying these ancient insights to twenty-first century addiction recovery is where I come in. I've been using the chi cycle as a therapeutic tool for my clients for a long time now, and they all notice significant improvements. Just by changing *when* they do things their energy levels improve; they become more productive, their skin and eyes become clearer, they lose weight (mainly a reduction in abdominal fat), cravings diminish and 'three-thirty-itis' disappears, as does emotional reactivity, insomnia and the dreaded pattern of always waking up alert at 3 am. But this is just the start. Where it gets really interesting, in terms of the chi cycle as a recovery lifestyle, is that doorways to altered states can also open up again.

Chi is the secret ingredient for a happy life,
and the chi-cycle is the recipe

LET'S GET MYSTICAL

Follow the chi-cycle recovery lifestyle and pretty much every amazing state you felt on drugs, from euphoria to enhancement to bliss, can be recaptured every day without drugs. Daoism is often called 'the art of intoxication' and, over time, following the chi cycle naturally delivers a series of intoxicating or altered states every day.

This kicks off with a connection to the mystical on waking, followed by knowing your cosmic self, going to work in an altered state, feeling peace at lunchtime and spending the early afternoon feeling stoned. After this comes some intergalactic travelling in a mystical meditation, 'forgetting' via creativity or sex, and then heading off on an overnight journey into astral chi. This lifestyle has to be every drug user's dream.

The part that is every drug user's nightmare, however, is the routine and discipline necessary to generate all those altered states. Each twenty-four hour cycle has a yang part (until lunchtime), and a yin part (until midnight). The idea is to align your activities with these great cosmic cycles. Basically, this means always doing productive active things in the yang time – the morning – and always doing laid-back things in the yin time – the afternoon and evening. You follow a daily routine that never shifts. This might sound boring, but in my mind it's nowhere near as boring as what happens if you quit drugs but keep your old random drug lifestyle.

Get high without drugs

THE RELAPSE CYCLE

A typical drug lifestyle is the opposite of aligned: you sleep in, drag yourself though the morning, come alive after lunch, then try to be productive late in the day because you got nothing done in the morning. You are being yin while the cosmos is yang, and vice versa. You are going against the flow and wasting energy. This builds the acquired self, increases your pain and misery and, if stick with this lifestyle after drugs, it encourages cravings and relapses.

It's perfectly understandable why people become unaligned. While you sleep you return to your cosmic self and are free from the acquired world and physical and emotional pain while you sleep. The minute you wake though, reality hits. Drifting back into sleep is very tempting, as is seeking an immediate distraction from your feelings, like listening to music, watching TV or having coffee and a cigarette. But starting the day like this puts you in a position of weakness and vulnerability. The mundane acquired world and other people's opinions will have too much power over you. You'll start thinking about drugs, and how they can make all that disappear. The drug parrot perches on your shoulder.

You probably won't want breakfast, because the thought of eating (let alone eating wholesome foods) is about as appealing as the idea of gnawing on some old cardboard. So you either skip it, choose coffee and cigarettes – which temporarily create the impression of movement but increase your underlying imbalances – or detonate the 'toxic-bomb' of sweet processed foods. Sugar creates a temporary sense of 'movement' and wheat makes you feel full, seeming to counter stagnation and emptiness, but you have just fed your acquired self and your irritation, frustration and emotional fragility. You have also topped-up your toxins, which intensifies your feelings of being stuck.

You won't feel like doing anything productive, so the stagnation increases. Everything around you becomes extremely annoying. You're missing something; you try more coffee, cigarettes and sugary snacks. That drug parrot is now squawking in your ear. The day drags towards a close, but you're not really tired, so you stay up late, watching TV or wandering around online. And, when you finally go to bed, you sleep poorly. So the next morning it's even harder to get up and get going. You feel heavy, lethargic and depressed, again. As the day progresses, it all gets slightly worse.

As there seems no escape from this downward cycle; you're ripe for a relapse and the parrot is probably out scoring for you now. I've seen this situation over and over again – the relapses that is, not the scoring parrots (that, I'd like to see). All the clients I treat who think they are diseased or losers because they keep relapsing, have this unrewarding, chi-depleting, unaligned lifestyle.

Reward yourself to avoid relapse

THE LAST RELAPSE

Relapsing is the natural outcome of following the normal Western lifestyle. But once you get the chi-cycle aligned lifestyle going, relapsing is no longer an issue. Chi experiences keep getting better, making drug experiences comparatively dirtier and madder than you expected. It can take a while to make the transition to chi, so don't be too hard on yourself if you do relapse. Most people quit via a relapse or two. I could write a whole book on my own relapses, but it would be a bit repetitive. Every chapter would start and finish the same way, except for the last one when I discovered chi.

My last relapse was a joint, although I didn't consider it a relapse at the time as, once you've been a speed addict, you don't consider marijuana to be a real drug. It was to be a reward for not doing drugs for so long and for working hard on my college studies. I'd gotten hold of a legendarily potent strain of cannabis and, as it had been a few years since I'd had hard drugs, I was fully expecting to recapture that great dreamy, chilled-out state that marijuana used to deliver in the good old pre-speed days.

But when I inhaled, nothing happened; it just felt toxic. The magic was gone. At the time I was puzzled; I had been living a really healthy lifestyle and it should have gotten me back into good shape for a drug high, but it hadn't. After spending so many years trying to give up drugs, it seemed the drugs had now given up on me. At the time I put it down to just another weird drug thing, but it stuck in my mind, the way significant things do. I had been doing chi practices for years by then and I now see that the chi states I was achieving had cancelled out the action of the drug. I had upgraded my source of energy, consciousness and information, and it overwrote the old programming.

Cravings are for an extraordinary life

REWARDS VS RELAPSE

The chi-cycle lifestyle creates a sense of being constantly rewarded, so it displaces the old association of drugs with reward. Because it is a lifestyle, it also gives you something to do all day so you won't be spending all your new drug-free time sitting around chatting to the parrot about how good drugs were, or would be again.

Additionally, aligning with the cycle allows a natural detox to occur every twenty-four hours. Every morning, the cosmic forces and your body can naturally work together to cleanse the toxins that make you feel stagnant, bloated, negative and emotionally weak. Moving and being productive until lunchtime also creates beneficial stress which moves stagnant energy. Being asleep by 11 pm allows your liver cleansing action to get underway. Live every day like this and you'll not only avoid those expensive relapses, but you will save on detoxes.

I've done the drug lifestyle and the chi lifestyle and I can tell you; aligning, feeling rewarded and being able to escape reality whenever you want is way better than being trapped in the limited acquired world. Every day on earth holds awesome unlimited possibilities. You don't want to waste a single day bogged down in emotional minefields, watching your health deteriorate and your purpose, happiness and sense of meaning slip away. You'll end up thinking that life sucks, and it really doesn't. Follow the chi cycle and stay in touch with your cosmic self instead. I believe that we all want to do this. I would go so far as to say we all *have* to, because our real business here on earth is to evolve our souls, but more on that later.

> *Your real business here is to evolve your soul*

RECOVERY TO DISCOVERY

On a purely practical level, this chi-cycle recovery lifestyle suits the massive new drug-using demographic, which is invisible and socially integrated. Some of this demographic do drugs on occasion, and can take it or leave it. Others choose to go about their daily business; school, work or socialising, on drugs – as this is their preferred reality – but they can regularly chill-out off the drugs for days or weeks without cravings. And then there are the high-level, fully functioning users who work and interact effectively, but can't get through a day without drugs. Usually no one apart from their drug associates or dealers know about their drug use. I once treated two ice-addicts who had worked in the same office for years and neither had any idea of the other's drug use.

In my day, drug users looked liked outsiders, behaved like outsiders and were treated as such. Generally speaking, we were part of a subculture that was disapproved of, and rejected by the mainstream population. Most of my friends remained marginalised or left town in an attempt to quit and make a new life elsewhere.

Drug users are no longer a subculture or a minority. They can't all up and leave town – it would be a global exodus. Even if they could, the 'leaving town' method of quitting hinges on being able to go somewhere where you can't get drugs, and not many places fit that description now. Even in the 1980s, when I travelled all the way from Germany to Australia, despite the fact that I knew no one in the country, it wasn't long before I was scoring drugs again.

The chi-cycle recovery lifestyle allows you to stay where you are and keep on doing what you usually do, because you don't have to get away from drugs if you have no interest in drugs. If you are taking drugs because you prefer a more interesting reality (and I believe all drug users do), but don't have a means of return to altered states, you'll just crave drugs. But aligning with the chi cycle allows you to quit successfully, because you'll have something to look forward to every day.

You will also tap into your destiny. According to the Daoists we all have a destiny, something we signed up to do here on earth. This is known as your 'contract with heaven'. Understanding what this is makes your life feel purposeful. This is a big deal indeed in terms of drug recovery. Walking blandly through life is not a satisfactory future for the explorers of the extraordinary. You need to burn with purpose. So, health and happiness, free altered states, a natural detox, getting on track to destiny and finding your cosmic self – it's not a bad deal in return for rearranging your daily schedule.

The chi cycle was a concept that intrigued me from the first time I came across it, particularly the references linking it with destiny, heavenly contracts and cosmic quests. But I had no idea of its true transformational potential until I lived it. I tuned into where my chi was during the day and recorded how various activities felt when aligned with different times. The results were outlined in my book *The Perfect Day Plan*, which revealed what to do every two hours of the day to enhance specific organ functions and create health and happiness.

But in the recovery context, we are focusing on the mystical, altered states aspect of the chi cycle and will be following the daily cosmic flow of yin and yang rather than two-hour segments. The goal is to initiate invisible internal processes which automatically generate altered states. You can't see any of this happen, but, as your drug use has sensitised you to the inner workings of chi, your organs and your cosmic connection, you can feel it. The more aligned you get your life, the more 'right' everything feels. Follow this feeling.

Make your lifestyle mystical

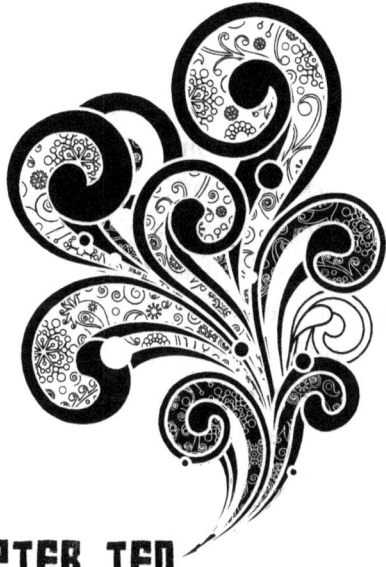

CHAPTER TEN
YANG TIME

Aligning with the chi cycle begins in the morning. Get up as early as you can and immediately do some chi practices and exercise. This gets chi moving and puts you in an altered state. This is exactly how you want to start each day after drugs. The alternative is starting out feeling stuck and trapped in normal reality – and that will make you want drugs. Having an extraordinary life – or not – after drugs, hinges entirely on how early you can get up and into chi each day. Early morning offers exclusive access to an assortment of mystical opportunities from downloading chi to getting on track to your destiny.

The details of your contract, your destiny, are coded and stored in your organs and you need to be in an altered state to access the information. This is why those trippers take peyote and wander around the desert on a vision quest. But if you hit an altered state naturally via a chi practice early in the morning, your internal organ code-breakers will naturally be activated, enabling information on your contract to be released. As this happens within the structure of the chi cycle it is in alignment with Dao, and other mystical processes are also activated. There are invisible destiny gateways available to keep you on the cosmic track throughout each day, and the first of these will now open. So you'll have some extraterrestrial help on your quest.

In the early morning, you also have the perfect internal organ environment for resolving the drug darkness and switching over to the light. Cosmic yang is gaining momentum at this time too, and just being up and moving means the force will be with you for the day ahead, so you won't be wasting your own reserves of chi. Get up early, do a chi practice and you will start out with a range of physical and metaphysical advantages.

Get a metaphysical start every day

THE COSMIC CHI CONNECTION

Cosmic chi also showers the earth early in the morning. If you do specific breathing techniques and chi practices at this time, you can access this. Remember, the more chi you have, the more extraordinary everything will become. Specific chi techniques are necessary to assist in this process. They can awaken cosmic chi, which can then find the cosmic self and draw it into your body.

Start with a classic Chi-gung. Stand still, arms by your sides, legs shoulder width apart and knees slightly bent. This is known as a 'correction posture'. It is a simple pose, but it aligns the three major energy centres in your body with Dao. Your analytical, judgmental internal dialogue (I'm a loser, I'm a hopeless addict, I can't do it etc.) automatically slows down, so you can get closer to your cosmic self. Then direct your awareness inwards to your five major organs (lungs, heart, liver, kidney and spleen) and outwards to the far reaches of the cosmos. This makes a connection between your organs and the cosmic chi matrix.

Then, while exhaling, squat down low and visualise scooping up earth energies with your hands. As you rise up, inhale and draw those energies to your heart with your hands. While still inhaling reach your arms up and then draw 'heavenly' energies down into your heart while exhaling. Repeat this slowly for several minutes. This simple action acknowledges that we belong equally in the physical and mystical worlds. Next I recommend doing a stationary Chi-gung, which 'gathers chi', followed by postures which circulate and direct that chi through your body. Chi heals, so this is the perfect time to direct chi to emotional or physical pain. After chi practices do some weights and cardio exercise.

Not many people like to get up early to do a chi practice (not even me and I've been doing it for decades), but once you are up and into it, it feels so good you won't want to stop. So think of it this way: if you once got up for drugs, as I did, you've already programmed yourself to wake up and change the way you feel. Keep doing that, but do it early in the morning and for chi highs. Not as much fun as getting up for drugs you say? Suck it up, because if you get up to find your cosmic self, eventually you are going to have more fun than you ever imagined.

Wake up to change the way you feel

FEED YOUR COSMIC SELF

We are after as many heightened states as possible each day after drugs, and also aiming to get ever closer to our cosmic side. Breakfast plays a critical support role in this. Sit down, relax and eat a warm cooked breakfast. This allows the mystical internal processes you initiated with the chi practices to continue. The awareness of your cosmic self will move to your heart, the seat of knowledge and love. The most common thing I hear from clients is 'I don't know who I am' or 'I'm nobody'; this chi-cycle lifestyle creates a powerful connection to who you really are and this becomes stronger every day.

But you need to eat breakfast for this. I treat plenty of people who tell me that they don't eat breakfast, as if it's a choice! It's not. Skip breakfast and you are reducing your chances of finding your cosmic self, and of being able to escape reality. A nourishing breakfast also provides the fuel for a productive morning so you won't be exploiting your own reserves of chi. Porridges or congees are ideal.

Most ex-users can't stomach food in the morning, let alone warm cooked food, but if you think 'yuck' just at the thought of this, it is an indication of nutrient and chi deficiency. High-powered nutritional supplements will help with this.

Think of cooking as an opportunity for alchemy. You can work with the elements – fire and chi – to create meals that support your cosmic quest. A certain amount of the chi of food is in the steam, and if you want the full chi-building mystical breakfast experience, take a moment before eating to allow the steam/chi to enter your meridians via an acupuncture point at the end of your nose. Its metaphysical role is to welcome your food. This might sound poetic, but Chinese medicine is highly practical. Expanding your awareness to consciously welcome your breakfast also improves your digestion – a critical factor in accelerating your drug recovery.

After a breakfast like this, you are now primed for some mystical visualisations and affirmations. There is a powerhouse meridian which runs all the way from your eyebrows, over the top of your head down your back, to your toes. It connects all the major organs. So, after you finish eating, sit still for a few minutes and visualise power rolling up that meridian – up your spine from the base, over the top of your head and down the centre of your forehead to the point of your third eye. This is the acupuncture point for clairvoyance (clear vision). Now project your intent for the day with the affirmation, 'I will see everything in the day ahead through the eyes of my cosmic self'. This gets your body, mind and spirit on the same page and ready to work hard.

Remember who you really are

GO TO WORK IN AN ALTERED STATE

Conjure up a past ice, speed or cocaine experience to get an idea of just how good an aligned morning's work can naturally feel. If you've started your day in chi, body and spirit, instead of waking up and letting your mind run riot, your mind can now be governed by your organs. It will be working for you. It will be a friend, rather than an enemy of Dao. As some information on your purpose and destiny has been released, your mind can now be harnessed to executing your cosmic goals.

Work hard now and you'll feel the exhilarating rush as your mind, chi and the cosmos move forward in unison. Your spleen and heart are being charged with cosmic chi now. As your spleen is connected to your mind, focus, clarity of thought and fluid communication, and your heart is the seat of intelligence and love, together they can light the 'fire of destiny'. It is our duty to pursue our destiny and dreams, but it's a duty we mostly neglect because we get caught up in the acquired world, and notions of being responsible, and doing what we are *supposed* to do rather than what we were *born* to do. 'It's too risky' is the mantra of the acquired self. This is not the path to happiness.

It doesn't matter how good a chi practice makes you feel, if you don't pursue your destiny as well, cravings will rise again. There's no point staying in a job that you used to be able to do on drugs or while hungover from drugs. Challenge yourself, expand your business into new areas, change your job, or train to be what your cosmic self longs for. This will probably trigger fear of failure or of the unknown, but keep moving forward regardless and you will build your willpower and strength. I believe that drugs are an evolutionary tool. Their role is to create change. Respect this by leaving the old behind and embracing the new in every part of your life. Be proactive and 'nourish' your destiny.

Use this yang time of the day to make a start on achieving your dreams. If you don't know what these are grab a piece of paper and divide it into two columns. Write in the left-hand side anything you can think of that you always wanted to do – whether it's starting a charity, writing a book, saving the rainforest or making a documentary. Then, in the right-hand column, list the steps necessary to practically achieve this; things like taking classes, studying scripts, applying for jobs or building your website. Do these tasks in the mornings.

You want each morning to feel purposeful and productive, otherwise you'll sense that something is wrong, something is missing. You don't know what it is so you'll think it's the drugs. Cravings arise making you susceptible to relapse.

So even if you have a job you don't like or consider meaningless, still work hard and purposefully until lunchtime. This moves stagnant chi, which means that making positive changes will become easier. Resist spending the morning gossiping at the water cooler or sending joke emails around. You won't be in sync with the cosmic forces and it will work against you.

If you are unemployed, avoid watching TV, lying around listening to music, reading magazines or doing things for entertainment in the morning. Unemployment means you have a fantastic opportunity to make finding your cosmic self your job (this is, in fact, everyone's real job). So during the morning look for books, websites or videos about inspiring people, challenging journeys, amazing superfoods, multidimensional universes, martial arts or cutting edge holistic therapies. Chi will flow.

Bear in mind that your life won't suddenly be easy once you follow your destiny. The path to purpose is never smooth, but it's not supposed to be. The idea is to just get stuck into it regardless. Getting involved with life on earth is how the Dao realises itself. We are here to do things, to have a go, and to do that in the yang part of the day with the backing of the cosmos.

Pursue your destiny

PEACE FOR LUNCH

There is a system behind an aligned day. Yang is expansion, it rises. Cosmic yang slowly builds in the first half of the day and if your actions have been aligned

with this – a chi practice, followed with a nourishing breakfast and at least four hours of working purposefully – information about your cosmic self will also rise and subtly infiltrate your consciousness. Lunchtime is an opportunity to experience the deep inner peace that the emotional security of a strong sense of self and purpose creates. This is a priceless feeling for an ex-drug user.

By lunchtime, cosmic yang switches over to yin and your actions need to align with this. Sit back and calmly eat a warm nourishing lunch. Again, what and how you eat is critical, because you will either be feeding your acquired self, depleting your chi and contributing to misery and confusion, or feeding your cosmic self, building chi and a bright future.

Having a sandwich at your desk, for example, or while rushing around multi-tasking, interrupts your inner mystical processes and feeds your acquired self. By 3:30 pm you'll be craving something like a sugar hit, a snooze or a line of Columbian marching powder. This interrupts your ability to know who you are and what you are here for and you'll be more likely to waste time doing acquired things like making other people's lives miserable or buying into other people's attempts to make your life miserable.

Feed your cosmic self with a warm nutritious meal though, and things will be different. The cosmic self is not interested in gossip, or in having opinions or judgment. It is free from reactive emotionality and accepts everything. The cosmic self doesn't look for value outside itself. The cosmic self doesn't eat sandwiches and it doesn't work through lunch. It understands how critical it is to live in harmony with the great cycles of yin and yang.

It is your duty to follow your dreams

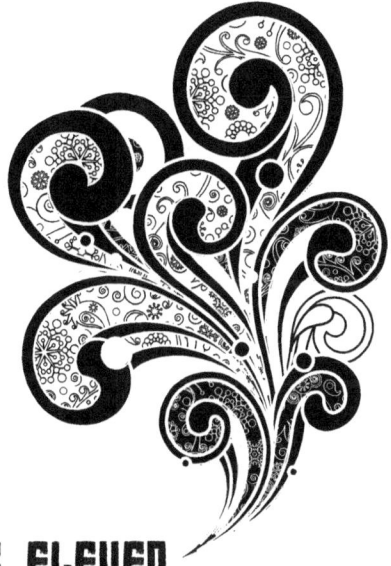

CHAPTER ELEVEN
YIN TIME

A good way to approach your afternoon is to imagine that you have smoked a big fat joint. You'd still be doing things, but not in such an outcome-oriented manner. Instead you'd have no opinion, you'd be cruising along. The goal for the afternoon is to sit back and roll with the yang momentum you built during the first half of the day. You want to capture that feeling of doing (yang) while being (yin).

Maybe you're now thinking well, why not just have a joint? But there's no need. In the hours after lunch the long meridian that we used for the morning's visualisation is being charged by cosmic chi. This meridian is loaded with acupuncture points that connect internally to all your organs but also externally to the chi matrix, so you have an opportunity to really feel cosmic connectivity. It creates a stoned sensation. Get aligned and tune in and you will feel this every afternoon for free.

Unfortunately, as most people's mornings are unproductive they have to start working hard *after* lunch in order to get everything done. The common response to my recommendation to 'sit back' in the afternoon is, 'that's not realistic'. But charging ahead in yang mode while the cosmos shifts into yin is what's not realistic here.

Do this, and you are no longer aligned and you'll be drifting off on your own. You will lose the sense of support, waste your energy and develop your acquired self. Sitting back is not about chilling-out, that would be unrealistic (chilling-out comes in later in the day). The idea is to keep working, but on less important things, as this harmonises your actions with the switch to cosmic yin.

The fundamental nature of existence is mystical and we are here to be mystical so being both energised and laid-back, and feeling stoned, is a realistic aim for the afternoon. Three-thirty-itis doesn't count as sitting back. If you are tired and lethargic and craving something, it is an indication that you have been exhausting your reserves of chi through an unaligned lifestyle. You are not missing chocolate, cigarettes, caffeine or drugs; you are missing support, belonging, connection and chi.

You are here to be mystical

TAKE A TRIP

After work, ideally somewhere around 6 pm, it is time to escape reality again, and 'roam the universe' in a magical meditation. Think of a favourite mind-blowing psychedelic drug experience to get an idea of what is on offer now. The Daoists have many different types of altered meditative states, but what we want to chase now is known as *Yuanyou*. It has been described as travel to distant realms and encounters with supernatural beings. It is an effortless meditative experience and, being a connoisseur of altered states, this is probably my favourite part of the day. I'd describe my experience of this meditation as the ultimate trip; a mash-up of the best parts of methamphetamine, marijuana, cocaine, mushrooms and heroin but with no side effects. Once you feel this state, all you want is to be there. Nothing else matters.

A day aligned with the chi cycle has prepared the internal organ states necessary to run this mystical meditation program (the morning chi practice is essential) so you just have to kick it off. Start by finding somewhere to be alone. Prepare by letting your face, the mask of your acquired self, relax and become expressionless, and set your intention.

I begin by saying 'Great Spirit, Father, Mother, God, Highest Source of Good (I like to cover all bases), please be with me and allow me to now receive my meditation'. Then I put my focus on the lower Dantian (the lower belly) and just hand over to Dao.

Instantly, the feeling from my morning Chi-gung returns in waves of ever-increasing intensity, building to an almost orgasmic finale. Cosmic chi is empowering your kidneys now, which are known as the 'mother of yin and yang'. And, while yin and yang merge in them, you can experience your true self in the midst of a merging of the cosmic creative forces. It is a mind-blowing trip. Afterwards I feel restored, refreshed and back in touch with my cosmic self. The yang activities of the day have been forgotten and now you can fully embrace yin.

Meditation takes you to the mystical

SEX AND THE CYCLE

As your kidneys store your sexual energy, this is also a good time for sex. One of the great attractions of being high on drugs is forgetting the obligations and limitations of the mundane world. Sexual experiences can deliver this state too. As sexual feelings intensify, yin and yang merge and you get that fantastic body–mind integration. You're not lying there analysing anything, you're not thinking 'hmm, now I need to move my leg two inches to the right, and my left arm up above my head', or 'maybe I'll Google that next position'. You don't follow the instructions of your mind; you are driven by chi.

If you are a yang type, you are probably thinking 'oh great, I can have sex every day at 6 pm'. Think again. Having a healthy sex life is very important. In Chinese medicine 'healthy' means not only at the right time but also the right amount; too much sex can deplete your chi, but not enough sex can drain your spirit. How much is beneficial is different for everyone, depending on factors including your constitutional type, age and health. But in most instances doing it every day is not considered beneficial. Following the chi-cycle lifestyle sensitises you to the forces of yin and yang so you naturally develop the ability to manage the yang drive for excessive sex.

Although imbalances such as the insatiable urge that leads to sex or porn addiction are common after drugs, so is the opposite condition of low libido or no sex drive. Loss of libido is considered to be sexual dysfunction in Western medicine, but in Chinese medicine it, and erectile issues for men, arise from chi deficiency and depletion. Impotence can be a strategy implemented by your body to preserve your chi for your major organ functions; like keeping your heart beating (which is why, for men, using performance enhancing drugs in these situations can be dangerous for your heart). Building chi is the solution for this and for low libido.

Another common post-drug condition is the inability to have 'normal sex' because after spectacularly intense drug-fuelled sex, sometimes for days on end, normal sex just feels mechanical. Prolonging states of heightened awareness is definitely the right idea in sex (and life in general), but doing so through drugs is not sustainable. The good news is that following the chi-cycle lifestyle, in conjunction with a medicinal diet, Chinese herbs and treatments (nutrients are critical here) can correct sexual imbalances, give you the control to prolong intense states and, ultimately, enable you to access cosmic chi during sex. Merging with the mystical in this way is a truly mind-blowing experience. No drug sex can ever match this. Forget the earth moving; you'll feel the cosmos move!

Chi prolongs heightened states

COSMIC CREATIVITY

Pleasure benefits chi, and enjoying yourself after you finish the day's work is an important part of the chi cycle. You can't have sex every day so you need some other pleasure options. This can be tricky after enjoying extraordinary drug states.

A lot of mainstream rehab programs and publications are now recommending enjoyable or fun activities in recovery. Some suggestions that I have come across recently include, 'dancing, even if there is no music' (not even worth discussing) and 'buying yourself a new pair of shoes' (seriously?). I've treated clients who tried parachuting, heli-skiing or drift-dives, but even these adrenalin-fuelled activities didn't do anything for them after drug highs, so I really don't think shoe shopping is going to cut it.

One of the most useless 'how to have fun after drugs' recommendations I have come across though, was the suggestion that you go to parties but instead of getting trashed, 'find pleasure in staying sober, talking to people and really getting into the conversation.' Dream on! Firstly, if you've quit drugs and are at a party, it's probably against your will as you'd rather be at home by yourself online or watching TV, because mixing with normal people makes you realise that there is something wrong with you, and secondly, being expected to enjoy talking to people who are probably all busy getting tanked is just ridiculous.

Expecting activities that might have been fun in your pre-drug days to be so again after drugs will just lead to disappointment. This will contribute to depression, cravings, relapse and, if you seek help for this, medication. Medical professionals view the inability to feel excitement or pleasure as depression, and mood-altering medication as the answer. But, as every drug user knows (except maybe the dedicated dope-smokers), what goes up must come down, and this applies to all mood-altering drugs, whether they are legal or illegal.

In Chinese medicine, the inability to feel pleasure or excitement is the result of depleted chi. There's nothing wrong with you. Following the chi-cycle recovery plan will gradually change this. Meanwhile shift your pleasure goals from doing something fun (nothing legal is going to be fun for you) to a creative pursuit, something that you can lose yourself in. We are always either 'acquired' or 'cosmic', there is nothing in between. So in that state of losing yourself, you are forgetting your acquired self and you are remembering or finding your cosmic self.

When I mention being creative to clients, most immediately say that they can't draw or sing, or whatever. But you don't have to be good at it; you just want to be immersed in it. You don't have to whip up a watercolour or write odes to flowers; there's plenty of great software for creating music, film or art projects. I mess around with making electronic music every night and it takes me right away from everything.

This is not the time to be practising scales, learning new programs, doing night classes or anything that requires concentration, because that means you are engaging with yang energies in a yin phase of the day and, as we all know by now, that's a big no-no. Fierce concentration belongs in the morning. If you do this in the evening you're no longer aligned and are more likely to be heading back to drugs.

After some creative activity it is the best time for an evening meal. Eat warm and nourishing, easily digestible foods that will support yin. Avoid processed foods, caffeine, wheat and sugar in the evening, at all costs. These are yang, heat-inducing substances that will feed your acquired self and impair your ability to fall asleep, the ultimate yin activity.

Shift from the fun of the senses to the joy of chi

SLEEP AND THE SOUL

Cosmic yin has been steadily increasing and by 9 pm 'astral chi' begins entering the earth's atmosphere. Astral chi has a dreamlike quality; it feels supportive and mystical. This feeling intensifies and peaks at midnight, the most yin time of the twenty-four hour cycle. Lots of ex-drug users like to be awake and doing things late at night, they have become what I call astral-chi junkies. If you have an unaligned lifestyle, you miss out on mystical connections throughout the day, you are cut off from Dao and feel incomplete and, desperately hungry for chi, for mystery and for something beyond normal, you seek the feeling of connection and support from astral chi.

But astral chi is there to support the journey into sleep. Being awake and/or working at night 'robs harmony' as the Daoists would say. Ideally you want to fall asleep between 9 pm and 11 pm, as cosmic chi floods your san jiao (the invisible organ) during this time, switching your operating system over from day chi to astral chi. Then the grand cosmic altered state finale can get underway while you sleep.

From 11 pm to 3 am, as cosmic chi activates your liver and gallbladder in turn, your soul travels home to the astral spheres. It receives guidance on your destiny from your spiritual mentors and soul family, and also the courage for you to follow your path.

At 3 am, as cosmic chi moves to your lungs, your soul returns to your body (if you always wake at 3 am it means you don't have the yin for this to be a smooth transition). By 5 am, as cosmic chi activates your large intestine (the organ which is responsible for getting rid of the old to allow the new in) you can maximise the benefits of your soul's overnight spiritual fact-finding mission, by doing your chi practice. Information on your destiny is released from your organs and the destiny gateways appear to guide you through another day. Each day your knowledge of who you are and what you are here for becomes stronger.

This is a fantastic, cosmically holistic, health and happiness system. But you need to sleep at night for it to work. And now we hit a hurdle. Sleep is the ultimate yin activity, but an unaligned life of not switching from yang to yin in the second half of the day, and overstimulating the senses means that your mind and soul, which are supposed to be feeling snug and comfy in their organ homes, can't settle and they become restless wanderers. You lie there awake.

I treat people who will wake up during the night to check their phone and answer texts or emails. This is mystical self-sabotage. Communication devices are awesome inventions, but they are yang tools, which belong to the productive hours of the day. So as you head off to bed imagine that you first have to pass through a mystical security gate, and put all that stuff in a tray to be held for you overnight.

You can do a brief Chi-gung to counter yang stimulation and help yourself fall asleep. Start by standing beside your bed in the same posture you used in the morning – arms by your sides, legs shoulder-width apart and knees slightly bent – to align the three major energy centres in your body with Dao. This also aligns your meridians and acupuncture points with the stars. Try to move from perceiving with your senses to perceiving with chi. Next, sit down on the side of the bed and immerse yourself in the feeling of infinity opening up as astral chi surrounds you. Then lie down on your back momentarily, with your arms crossed over your chest, over your heart chakra (doing the Dracula), and once you feel the drift sensation, move into the recommended sleep posture.

Lie on your right side, with your legs slightly bent and resting in front of the pillow and your left arm resting on your left thigh. This puts your heart in an elevated position, which means that blood can circulate freely, and your liver in a low position which means that blood can collect there (your liver cleanses your blood overnight). Your stomach is also in a position that facilitates the downward movement of food. Then let the cosmos take over and carry your soul home.

Sleep is the most cosmic, mysterious and magical part of the entire twenty-four hours, and the part where you get to effortlessly return to your cosmic self. And the best bit – all you have to do is lie back, shut your eyes and think of the cosmos!

Set your soul free

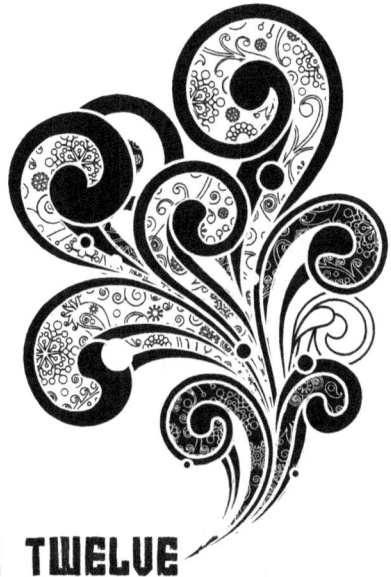

CHAPTER TWELVE
ONE COSMIC DAY

One mainstream recovery concept I do like is living one day at a time. Make it a day aligned with the chi cycle and then repeat it as many times as possible for the rest of your life. As you've probably noticed by now, alignment will entail major change from a day in the old drug lifestyle. So don't jump up at the crack of dawn the day after quitting drugs and then try to align your entire life with the chi-cycle.

Just getting out of bed might be a major challenge, so focus on nutrient therapy first and work towards having three nutritious meals a day. Take little steps towards establishing parts of the routine when you can. For example, you could begin doing some gentle exercises or Tai-chi later in the day when you feel more up to it, rather than early in the morning. Once you get a rhythm established, then move towards alignment.

Have a no-rule day once a week, so that you don't feel trapped by routine. Sleep in, eat whatever you want, break the routine, but always in a way in which you are able to 'return' the following morning (so no forty-eight hour drug or booze benders). Over time your no-rule day activities will become milder (6 am is a sleep-in for me now). The more chi you build, the more your sense of purpose and happiness increases. You'll start wanting more of that and will naturally avoid activities that have a negative impact on this.

Turn the psychedelic revolution into
psychedelic evolution

STICK WITH THE PROGRAM

Your mind will probably still be in 'enemy of Dao' mode when you begin your lifestyle shift. You won't believe how many excuses it will come up with for staying in bed or skipping breakfast or generally avoiding the process of finding your cosmic self. Time and time again I see people quit drugs, take up the chi cycle, begin to feel change and then suddenly reject it. They tell me it's not for them or the Tai-chi teacher was a loser, the gym sucked or everyone in the health food store was a weirdo, or they find some other reason to give in to the old acquired habits. This is a normal part of the process, and every time you make yourself get back on path you build your willpower and chi.

People around you are not going to be living with the chi cycle either, so keep in mind that you'll have to overcome not only your own resistance, but also social pressure. Long before I knew about chi, I'd realised that I needed a tightly scheduled health-focused lifestyle just to stay sane and functional. So I refused to ever shift from my routine for anything. This created ongoing friction with family and friends. I was accused of being a fitness freak, of being antisocial or difficult. Unbelievably, one close relative who'd spent years telling me what a drugged-out loser I was, actually told me that I was more fun on drugs.

But after I quit drugs I simply couldn't afford to follow the random lifestyle of the normal world. No ex-user can – ever. We need to live in a very different way. I wasn't able to explain any of that back then though, so all I could do was say 'no'. Turns out I got that right. Even back in ancient times, the Daoist sages saw how damaging trying to fit in with social expectations could be to an individual's health and happiness. Their solution was to say 'no'. This is considered to be one of the most powerful ways to build chi. Since you've broken all the rules already, you are in a great position to say 'no' to social expectations that will make it impossible or difficult for you to stick to your chi-building lifestyle.

While you're at it, say 'no' to the things that make you want to do drugs too. Try not to watch movies or listen to music that makes drug use look cool and fun. This is tricky, as popular culture is saturated with drug references, but do your best. Don't hang out with your drug-using partying friends, or let them crash at your place, while you are fragile and prone to relapse.

Try saying 'no' to negative thoughts too. It will be tempting to become fixated on what is wrong with everything and everyone around you after you quit, but this is due to internal organ imbalances; it's not an accurate reading of the world. Counter this negative pull by seeking positive input of any sort that reinforces the idea of achievement through movement. Read or watch inspiring stories about people – sports stars, artists, activists – who achieve against the odds. Don't underestimate the power of this material and go for anything that works for you.

When I was going through the worst of my post-drug depression I used to watch the early *Rocky* movies. Rocky lived in a world of physical and emotional pain, and he faced resistance on every front, but he kept fighting. His drive to keep moving forward helped me hang on to that attitude in the face of my own overwhelming desire to give in. No one could understand why I kept watching those movies, but they didn't wake up each morning and immediately think of dying.

Everyone will have opinions on how you should be living and what you should be doing after drugs. But the more you align with the chi cycle and the more chi practice you do, the less influence this will have on you. In the *Dao De Ching*, Lao-tzu states that you don't need governance if you know the way from within. Chi-cycle alignment provides a set of guidelines to live by. It harmonises you with natural rather than man-made laws and, as a result, you will always act in a manner that is beneficial to yourself and others.

Saying 'no' is one of the most powerful ways to build chi

EVERYONE'S A WINNER

An aligned chi-building lifestyle is a win-win solution for everyone. It is well worth the relatively small discomforts of rising early and repeating a routine. And really, if you ever want to feel more than normal again, there are no other viable post-drug lifestyle options. The fun drugs have run their course; we've established that you can't go 'back to normal'; just being healthy and fit isn't enough and the other option, of being medicated for the rest of your life on non-fun drugs, is just as bad as being on recreational drugs (and you don't even get the highs).

But if everything you do, from getting up in the morning to going to bed at night, contributes to building chi, then everything feels a little more extraordinary every day. You will eventually start looking forward to the next day to continue this long slow high. So take it day by day.

Think of your recovery as a road trip in which you can't see your final destination, only the stretch of road ahead. Just as each section you travel reveals the next, each time you take the cosmic option to build chi – regardless of how small or insignificant it might seem – it will introduce a possibility, evoke a feeling, and connect you to something or someone. Every movement creates another, and all sorts of possibilities open up.

Extraordinary lives unfold one day at a time

HAPPILY EVER AFTER DRUGS

Begin this journey by rethinking your past from the perspective of everything you got right, including: prioritising your inner state, wanting to escape reality, exploring the mystical, rejecting social falseness, transcending limits, feeling enhanced and chasing your dreams. Then use chi as the medium to find your cosmic self.

Start your revision of your past from the second time you took drugs. My theory is that no one knows what's going to happen the first time; it's when you deliberately attempt to recapture what did happen, that it gets interesting. You might think you repeated drugs just for fun or 'for laughs', but when clients tell me that, I always point out that there are amusement parks for fun. These are much cheaper than drugs and remove the possibility of getting addicted and ruining people's weddings (yep, did that) or participating in illegal fundraising activities (yes again). For laughs, there are jokes or the option of chuckling away with your friends in front of sitcoms. But it's not quite the same, is it? If it was, you wouldn't be reading this book.

After decades in this business, I believe that the desire to repeat drug experiences comes from a longing for mystical connection. Accordingly, the term 'recreational' is misleading; contrary to popular opinion this is serious business that you have been engaged in. We are all familiar with that clichéd movie scene in which a character takes a mind-altering substance and, suddenly seeing the non-ordinary world open up in front of them, gazes around with an awestruck expression saying, 'Unreal, man'.

This is supposed to be comedy, but when you are high and see the universe expand, or love everyone unconditionally, or are able to listen to someone rambling on about nothing and be present, saying 'real, man' would be more appropriate, because something about your true cosmic nature has been revealed.

What everyone thinks of as unreal – the mystical world, the one concerned with destiny and spirit and soul – is the permanent one. What everyone accepts as being real – the material world – is, in fact, temporary. It is when we find ourselves believing that the acquired world and our jobs and endless emotional dramas constitute the full extent of reality, that we should look around and say, 'Unreal, man'.

Chi is the medium to find your cosmic self

UNREAL REALITY

If you were drawn to repeat a drug experience it was because that unreal version of reality was not enough

for you. It is not *supposed* to be enough. I wish I'd known this. I'd never felt satisfied with ordinary reality, even as a child. I dreamt of having special powers and of travelling to other dimensions, but I was regularly told I was a dreamer, and I should 'grow up' or 'get real'.

Everyone else seemed fine with ordinary reality, so I started thinking that there was something wrong with me. Valium numbed that sensation, which is why I took to it so quickly, but a few years later, when LSD and other mind-altering substances made everything I had dreamt of real, I saw that I had been right; the universe truly was a mystical, magical place.

Drugs were my escape route, and drug-altered states fast became my preferred reality. This is where I felt at home. But this was not because anything went wrong for me, but rather because 1970s suburban Germany, with its emphasis on material wealth, social status, external appearances and its obsession with what the neighbours thought, did not feel like home to me. The Daoists flagged this issue centuries back. They saw how believing that the material or acquired world is all there is, leads to misery and to 'not feeling at home on earth'. Every drug user I treat these days can relate to this.

It is the same fundamental longing for something more than ordinary that makes them resonate with drug states. All it takes is a line of coke, a happy pill or a joint and the most boring chore in the most mundane place becomes an amazing multidimensional experience. You're still 'here' interacting in the normal world, but it doesn't look or feel normal any more. This feels right because essentially, it is.

But keep using drugs, and you drift from Dao; your acquired self becomes stronger, as does the feeling of not being at home on earth. The acquired response is to find someone or something to blame for your alienation and pain. I ended up with the anarchists fighting street battles against the police and what we called 'the establishment'. But what I was really protesting against was the loss of my access to the mystical.

The chi-cycle lifestyle is a bridge from the mundane to the mystical. Resist the urge to give in, to live an acquired life and to take what seems to be the easy path. Do a daily chi practice, follow the cycle and make finding your cosmic self your priority, and you can cross that bridge at will. Then you will always know who you are and where you really belong. You will feel at home everywhere: in your body, your home and community, on the planet and in the cosmos. This is how reality should feel.

The fundamental nature of life is mystical

SOUL EVOLUTION

Finding your cosmic self is every drug users' responsibility. We usually see the words *drugs* and *irresponsibility* paired, but if you've taken drugs you have set something significant in train and I believe you have a responsibility to see it through. None of us are here on earth just for entertainment. Recreational drugs are powerful transformational substances, not a DIY fun-kit. Those of us that said 'yes' did not do so just to have fun.

We initiated a transformational process and now it's time to follow through.

The Daoists believe that we are here to evolve our souls. This process begins with awakening to the fact that there is something beyond the physical, followed by the desire to *feel* the connection to this. You have this underway because you already know that there is more than normal reality out there. You may have run into aliens, seen through walls or experienced telepathy. You understand that inexplicable things and invisible forces surround us. Your ongoing drug experiences were evidence of your desire to explore and feel this. Now just switch methods from drugs to chi practices.

I've been really pushing doing a chi practice because, if you make yourself do this every day, one day you will find yourself *wanting* to do it. Keep going, and then you start *having* to do it. You will naturally shift from feeling chi, to consciously moving and directing chi. This is known as 'chi cultivation'. This is the ultimate escape route.

You're already familiar with this process. When you take a drug, as soon as it hits your system it's – wow! You instantly take note of what is happening internally, this is you 'discovering' chi. Dancing on ecstasy, getting into the music, phoning all your friends, getting into sex, are all versions of 'directing' or 'circulating' chi. You work with these feelings until you hit the zone where everything is flowing, and you don't perceive yourself as a separate entity any more; you perceive yourself via everything around you – the music, the people. You feel totally connected with all there is. Your singular awareness dissolves into cosmic awareness. The universe reshapes itself around you.

This is exactly the chi sequence to pursue afterwards, of discovering, gathering, and directing chi. Your chi practice will then naturally take you towards the ultimate state of dissolving in chi. One day you will find you are no longer consciously moving through the postures and directing chi flow, you have become it. You've spontaneously shifted into a higher state and crossed the bridge to non-ordinary reality. Once you chase and crave chi states like you once craved drugs or alcohol, you have begun to live for your spirit as much as for the material world.

Drugs are an evolutionary tool

ALIGN WITH THE STARS

The third stage of soul evolution is what contemporary Daoist scholars call 'cosmicisation'. This is finding your cosmic self and becoming cosmically aligned. I've talked about the cosmic self a lot so far but there is a literal aspect to this concept.

In Chinese medicine, we come from the stars and we are connected to the stars (each acupuncture point in your body aligns with a star). Doing a daily chi practice aligns your body with the stars, and following the chi-cycle lifestyle aligns your life with the stars. When you feel equally at home with the stars as with your daily life on earth, you'll know you have achieved cosmicisation.

So, if you repeated a drug experience, you were chasing something mystical, spontaneous yet eternal – an experience of Dao. You were, in fact, all along, on a mystical quest, not just on drugs. Questing might sound like something from a fairytale, but the minute you become rational about your drug use and recovery, and start applying intellect and analysis, it takes the Dao, the creative spontaneity, out of the equation. Instead, continue your quest by working with the mystical cosmic forces, yin and yang and chi, and there are no limits.

Just trust that the mystical world is as real as the material world; trust in your chi practice, follow the chi-cycle recovery plan, and you will keep one foot in the mystical and one in the material world. You will find your cosmic self. This means you won't get caught up in emotionality or right and wrong. You will be able to hold onto the positives and see things as they really are. You will understand why you took drugs. You will have no regrets, feel no resentment and nothing will be unresolved. You will be fundamentally happy in everything you do, regardless of outcomes. You will see that we are all in the same boat, and you will begin to feel fortunate. This is true freedom.

Your drug journey might have broken you down physically, emotionally or spiritually, but if that becomes the catalyst for you to discover chi, cosmically reconnect through the chi cycle, and relaunch your mystical quest, be forever grateful, because everything is now in place for you to live happily ever after.

a t to e a t e t e as r 1

OTHER TITLES BY THIS AUTHOR

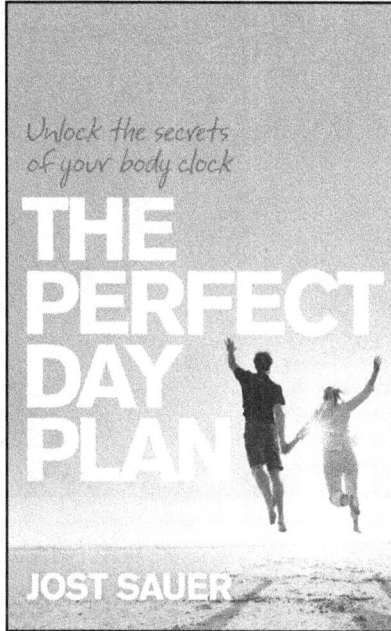

THE PERFECT DAY PLAN

In this first contemporary popularisation of the ancient Chinese chi-cycle, you will discover the best time to get up, to have sex, to have an argument, to eat, meditate and sleep. If you want a medicinal and magical lifestyle, this is the book for you.

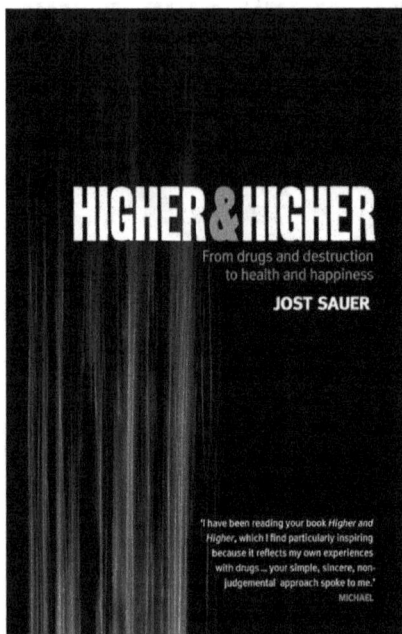

HIGHER AND HIGHER

Interweaving Jost's own experiences of speed-addiction with traditional Chinese medicine, this entertaining, uplifting and inspirational read, takes you on a roller-coaster ride from the hippie dream to the wellness industry. Described as 'Lao-Tzu meets Hunter S. Thompson', Higher and Higher shares insights into addiction, the human need to feel good, and ultimately offers everyone a sustainable path to the ultimate high.

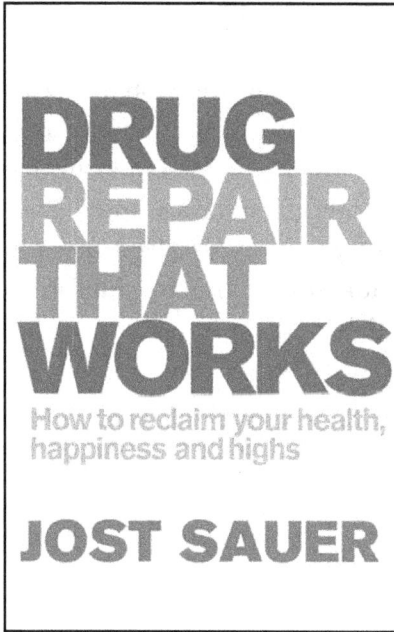

DRUG REPAIR THAT WORKS

Psychedelic, insightful, spiritual and practical, Drug Repair that Works is one of the most provocative books written about recreational drugs in recent times. Join Jost on a revelatory journey through the invisible worlds from addiction to psychosis to recovery. Prepare to abandon everything you thought you knew about recreational drugs.

ACKNOWLEDGMENTS

My thanks to Leon, Kylie and Conan Fitzpatrick for their valuable input. Thanks to my editor, Helena Bond, for helping this become a better book, to Tony Giacca for designing the cover I always wanted and to Elizabeth Jewel, editor of *Living Now Magazine*, for the ongoing support and for continuing to publish my sometimes outrageous articles.